Colour **Aids**

Dermatology

J. D. Wilkinson MB BS MRCP

Consultant Dermatologist, Wycombe General
Hospital, High Wycombe, UK

S. Shaw MB ChB MRCP

Associate Specialist in Dermatology, Wycombe
General Hospital, High Wycombe, UK

D. A. Fenton MB ChB MRCP

Senior Registrar in Dermatology, St Thomas's
Hospital, London, UK

Churchill Livingstone

EDINBURGH LONDON MELBOURNE AND NEW YORK 1987

CHURCHILL LIVINGSTONE
Medical Division of Longman Group UK Limited

Distributed in the United States of America by
Churchill Livingstone Inc., 1560 Broadway, New
York, N.Y. 10036, and by associated companies,
branches and representatives throughout the
world.

First published 1987
  Reprinted 1990

ISBN 0-443-02822-2

British Library Cataloguing in Publication Data

Wilkinson, J. D.
  Dermatology.—(Colour aids)
  1. Dermatology—Atlases
  I. Title II. Shaw, S. III. Fenton, D. A.
  IV. Series
  616.5'0022'2   RL81

Library of Congress Cataloging in Publication Data

Wilkinson, J. D.
  Dermatology.
  (Colour aids)
  1. Skin—Diseases—Atlases. 2. Dermatology—Atlases.
I. Shaw, S. II. Fenton, David A. III. Title.
IV. Series. [DNLM: 1. Dermatology—atlases.
WR 17 W687d]
RL81.W55 1987   616.5   87-762

Produced by Longman Group (FE) Ltd
Printed in Hong Kong

Acknowledgements

We would like to acknowledge the expert assistance of Alison Carter and Rosemary Ray, Department of Medical Illustration, Wycombe General Hospital. We also extend our thanks to the Department of Medical Illustration at The Radcliffe Infirmary, Oxford, for their permission to reproduce illustrations borrowed from their collection.

High Wycombe and London, 1987   J. D. W
                                                                    S. S.
                                                                  D. A. F.

Contents

Benign Childhood Pigmented Naevi (1)

Freckles (Fig. 1)

Aetiology
Increased activity of melanocytes.

Clinical features
Brown macules (usually in redheads). Appear in early childhood, and darken on sun exposure.

Lentigo

Aetiology
A localised proliferation of melanocytes.

Clinical features
Areas of brown or black pigmentation, usually 1–2 mm in diameter. Appear in childhood but may proliferate in adulthood. Do not darken or proliferate on sun exposure (Fig. 2).

Treatment
None. However, a solitary lentigo appearing in adult life and continuing to grow may be a malignant melanoma.

Pigmented naevus/birthmark (Fig. 3)

Aetiology
Developmental defect.

Clinical features
Localised pigmented and sometimes hairy naevus, present from birth, up to 2–3 cm in size. Giant hairy naevus is a rare developmental defect with a potential for malignant transformation. Surgical excision should be considered.

Treatment
None; excision if required.

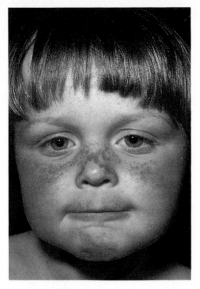

Fig. 1 Freckles.

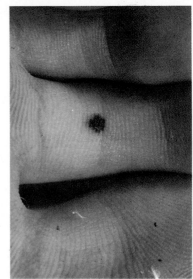

Fig. 2 Lentigo.

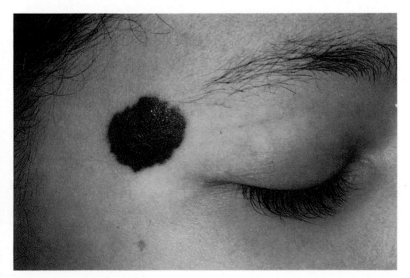

Fig. 3 Pigmented birthmark.

Cellular naevus

Synonym | Melanocytic/pigmented naevus or mole.

Aetiology | Developmental defect. Melanocyte proliferation at the dermo-epidermal junction or in the dermis.

Clinical features | Not normally present at birth, but develop during childhood, particularly at puberty. May enlarge or darken during pregnancy. Pink, brown or black, flat or raised, hairy or non-hairy (Figs. 4, 5). Blue naevus (Fig. 6) is a variant with dermal pigmentation. Malignant transformation is possible in those with large numbers of pigmented naevi or 'atypical' moles and a family history of melanoma.

Treatment | Excision only in the case of frequent trauma or malignant transformation. All excised moles should be submitted for histology.

Juvenile melanoma (benign)

Synonym | Spitz naevus.

Aetiology | A variant of cellular naevus.

Clinical features | A solitary, reddish-brown nodule occurring in childhood (usually affecting the face), growing rapidly to 1 cm. Benign, although the histology may resemble malignant melanoma (Fig. 7).

Treatment | None. Simple excision.

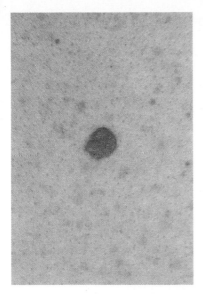

Fig. 4 Cellular naevus.

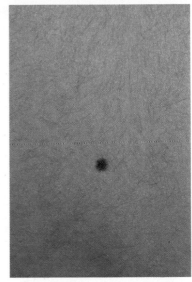

Fig. 5 Pigmented cellular naevus.

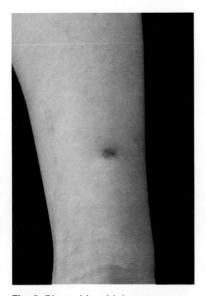

Fig. 6 Blue rubber-bleb naevus.

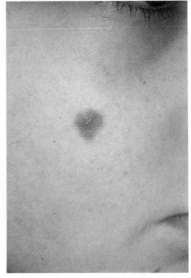

Fig. 7 Juvenile melanoma (Spitz naevus).

Genodermatoses (1)

Hereditary haemorrhagic telangiectasia

Synonym Rendu-Osler-Weber disease.

Aetiology Autosomal dominant inherited disorder.

Clinical features Telangiectasia of various sizes occur on the lips, face, ears, palms and soles. The mucous membranes of the lips, tongue and nose are frequently affected causing epistaxis; gastrointestinal tract involvement leads to haemorrhage and iron deficiency anaemia (Fig. 8).

Treatment Iron supplements may be required. Epistaxis can be treated with cauterisation.

Peutz-Jeghers syndrome

Synonym Periorificial lentiginosis.

Aetiology Rare autosomal dominant inherited disorder.

Clinical features Blue-brown macules affect the buccal mucosa, gums, lips, palate, palms and soles (Figs. 9, 10). Lentigines are obvious either at, or soon after birth. The condition is associated with small intestinal polyps. These may cause recurrent intersusception or ulcerate and lead to haemorrhage. Malignant transformation of polyps may occur but is rare.

Treatment The lentigines require no therapy.

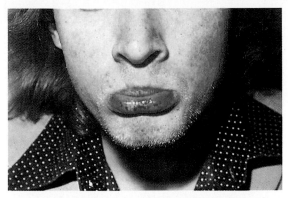

Fig. 8 Hereditary haemorrhagic telangiectasia.

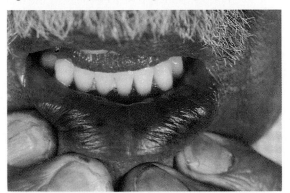

Fig. 9 Macular pigmentation of lips in Peutz-Jeghers syndrome.

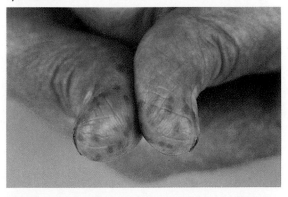

Fig. 10 Macular pigmentation of finger-tips in Peutz-Jeghers syndrome.

| # Genodermatoses (2)

Neurofibromatosis

Synonym   Recklinghausen's disease.

Aetiology   An autosomal dominant inherited condition with approximately 50% rate of new mutations.

Clinical features   Characterised by multiple, light brown, 'café-au-lait', macular patches of several cm diameter (Fig. 11). Some may be present from birth. There may also be axillary freckling (Fig. 12). The skin neurofibromas which develop as the child grow up are soft, dome-shaped, pedunculated or plexiform. They vary in number from a few to hundreds (Fig. 13). Size also varies from a few mm to enormous plexiform neuromas with hypertrophy of the subcutaneous tissues and skin. Systemic manifestations include kyphosis, scoliosis, bone cysts, phaeochromocytoma, acromegaly, acoustic neuroma, glioma and mental deficiency.

Treatment   Genetic counselling; excision of symptomatic neurofibromas.

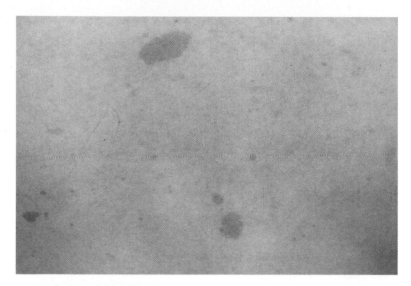

Fig. 11 'Café-au-lait' spots.

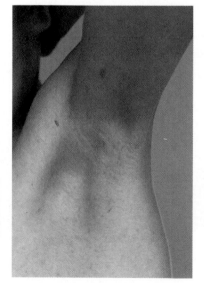

Fig. 12 Axillary freckling.

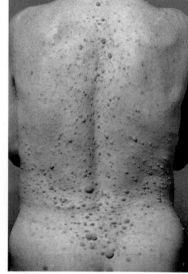

Fig. 13 Neurofibromatosis.

| # Genodermatoses (3)

Tuberous sclerosis

Synonym | Epiloia.

Aetiology | Autosomal dominant condition of skin and CNS.

Clinical features | Depigmented 'ash-leaf'-shaped macules occur on the trunk and limbs, varying in size from a few mm to a few cm. They may be more obvious under Wood's light (Fig. 14). There is no treatment. Other characteristic lesions present are as follows.

Clinical features | *Adenoma sebaceum*
Cutaneous angiofibromata produce small discrete pink papules affecting mainly the central face (Fig. 15). They are not present at birth but appear within the first few years of life. Can be confused with acne.

Treatment | Diathermy, dermabrasion or CO_2 or argon laser.

Clinical features | *Periungual fibromas*
Firm, smooth, filiform tumours emerging from the base of the nails (Fig. 16).

Treatment | None. Excision or diathermy.

Clinical features | *Shagreen patches* (collagen naevi)
Skin coloured/yellowish plaques occurring on the trunk.

Treatment | None.

Fig. 14 'Ash-leaf' spot.

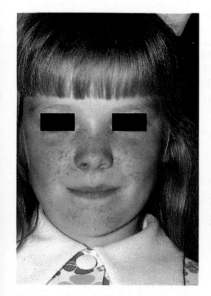

Fig. 15 Adenoma sebaceum.

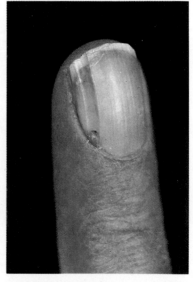

Fig. 16 Periungual fibroma causing distortion of nail plate.

Ehlers-Danlos syndrome

Aetiology

A rare group of inherited collagen disorders.

Clinical features

The skin is characteristically soft, doughy and hyperextensible, the joints are hypermobile or 'double-jointed' (Fig. 17). Cutis laxa may occur (Fig. 18). The skin is fragile and bruises easily; scars are atrophic and wide (Fig. 19). The sclerae are blue.

Treatment

No specific therapy, but lacerations/injuries require specialist attention to minimise scarring.

Pseudoxanthoma elasticum

Aetiology

Rare inherited disorder of elastic tissue.

Clinical features

Distinctive skin lesions, retinal changes and vascular disturbances. The skin is soft, lax and wrinkled with yellowish papules in a reticulate pattern or in plaques, giving the appearance of chicken skin or 'peau d'orange'. The sides of the neck, axillae and anticubital fossae are characteristically affected (Fig. 20). Slate-grey angioid streaks are seen on the retina. Arterial involvement may cause haemorrhage from the gut or elsewhere. Hypertension is also common.

Treatment

Avoid traumatic sports/hobbies or occupations which may lead to eye damage.

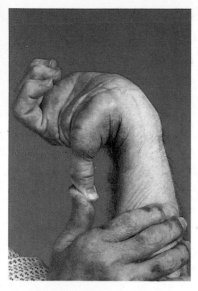

Fig. 17 Hyperextensible joint (Ehlers-Danlos).

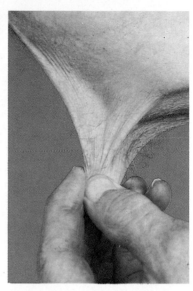

Fig. 18 Cutis laxa (Ehlers-Danlos).

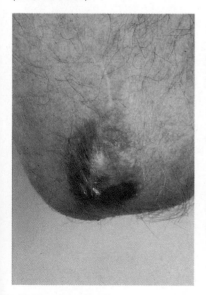

Fig. 19 Atrophic scar.

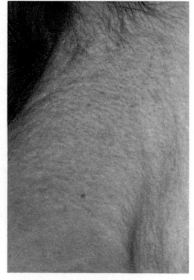

Fig. 20 Peau d'orange (PXE).

3 | Benign Childhood Vascular Tumours (1)

Portwine stain (capillary haemangioma)

Aetiology

Developmental defect of mature dermal capillaries.

Clinical features

An erythematous or purplish macular naevus (Fig. 21) present at birth. Usually unilateral, affecting face, trunk or limb, and variable in size. Possibly associated underlying arteriovenous malformation. Limb involvement may result in hypertrophy (Klippel-Trenauney syndrome); a capillary naevus in the trigeminal area may be part of the Sturge-Weber syndrome.

Treatment

Cosmetic camouflage; argon laser may help.

Strawberry naevus (cavernous haemangioma)

Aetiology

Developmental; benign angioblastic proliferation.

Clinical features

Develops rapidly during the first 6 months of life. A well-demarcated, compressible vascular swelling (Figs. 22, 23). Normally undergoes spontaneous resolution. Haemorrhage, ulceration and thrombocytopenia are rare complications.

Treatment

None. Spontaneous resolution. Surgery for redundant folds of skin. High dose steroids (rarely) given if severe thrombocytopenia, cardiac failure, or vital functions affected.

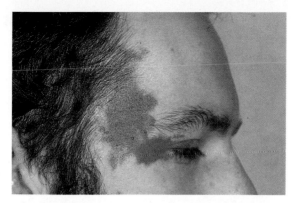

Fig. 21 Portwine stain.

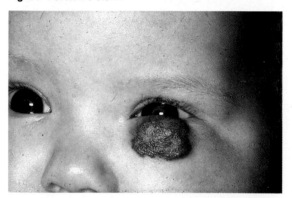

Fig. 22 Strawberry naevus.

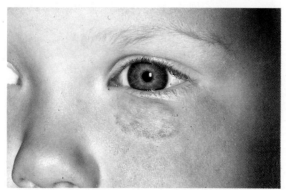

Fig. 23 Spontaneous resolution of same strawberry naevus.

Benign Childhood Vascular Tumours (2)

Spider naevus

Aetiology

A small, superficial arteriole giving rise to a localised telangiectasia.

Clinical features

A central, raised, erythematous papule with radiating dilated capillaries. If lesions are multiple and involve mucosal surfaces, hereditary haemorrhagic telangiectasia should be considered.

Treatment

'Cold-point' cautery or 'epilating' electrodiathermy to the cental arteriole.

Salmon patch

Aetiology

A localised, capillary, telangiectatic naevus.

Clinical features

A pale pink area, commonly found in newborn infants on the glabella or over one eye (Fig. 25). No treatment is required

Pyogenic granuloma

Aetiology

Abnormal proliferation of capillaries following trauma or infection.

Clinical features

A friable and often pedunculated vascular nodule, bleeding easily and profusely when traumatised.

Treatment

Curettage and cautery under local anaesthetic. In adults, histology is necessary: the lesion can be confused with amelanotic malignant melanoma.

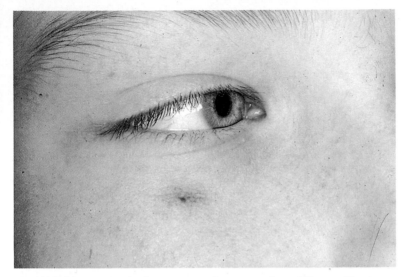

Fig. 24 Spider naevus. Lesions commonly occur on face. Often proliferate during pregnancy or liver disease.

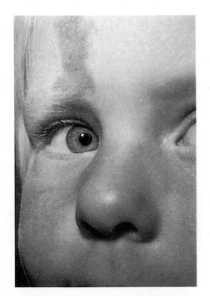

Fig. 25 Salmon patch. Facial lesions fade but those on nape of neck may persist.

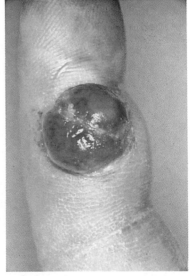

Fig. 26 Pyogenic granuloma. Grows rapidly, commonly affecting areas of trauma.

Napkin candidiasis

Aetiology

Yeast infection with *Candida albicans.*

Clinical features

Well-demarcated erythema with scaling extending from the perineum, normally involving the skin folds. There may be isolated 'satellite' lesions and/or pustules. Oral lesions and intertriginous infections are common (Figs. 27, 28) (see also p. 137).

Treatment

Swabs. Nystatin and imidazole creams (or a hydrocortisone/imidazole or antiseptic combination). Reduction of occlusion and eradication of yeast carriage. An appropriate dusting powder may prevent relapse.

Napkin psoriasis (Fig. 29)

Aetiology

Local factors; possible genetic predisposition.

Clinical features

Develops suddenly, normally at about 4–8 weeks. Dark-red and scaly lesions with well-defined margins in the napkin area and often on the scalp. Smaller scattered lesions can develop elsewhere on the trunk. Napkin area lesions are larger, asymptomatic and may extend to the flexures. Often clears spontaneously within a few weeks.

Treatment

Bland applications and mild topical steroids or steroid/antiseptic combinations.

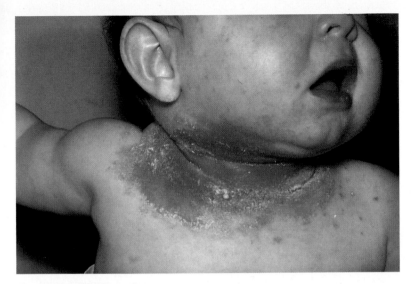

Fig. 27 Candidal intertrigo.

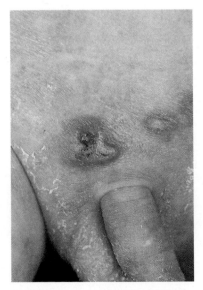

Fig. 28 Granuloma gluteale infantum (*candida*).

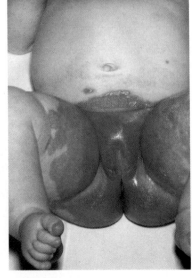

Fig. 29 Psoriasiform napkin rash.

Seborrhoeic eczema

Aetiology

Unknown. Constitutional and microbial factors may coexist.

Clinical features

Appearance at 2–10 weeks. Asymptomatic, well-defined, round or oval patches of erythema and greasy scaling extending to form gyrate patterns in the genitocrural flexures. Scalp, ears and other body folds may be involved (Fig. 30).

Treatment

Cleansing cream and mild topical steroid/antiseptic.

Napkin dermatitis

Aetiology

Inflammatory disorder produced by prolonged contact with urine, faeces or irritant chemicals in napkin. May be first manifestation of atopic eczema.

Clinical features

Genitalia, buttocks, lower abdomen and upper thighs are affected. Flexures are normally spared (Fig. 31). Initial erythema, but vesicles, papules, erosions and ulcers may develop. Fine scaling with glazed erythema is seen in chronic forms.

Treatment

Emollients and weak topical steroids. Frequent changing and thorough cleaning with a mild non-soap cleanser. Plastic napkins/pants should be avoided and nappies left off where possible. A barrier cream can be used at night. Candidiasis or secondary bacterial infections should be treated appropriately.

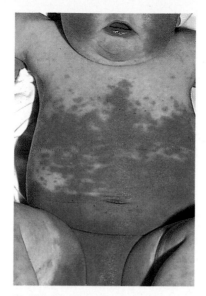

Fig. 30 Seborrhoeic dermatitis of infants.

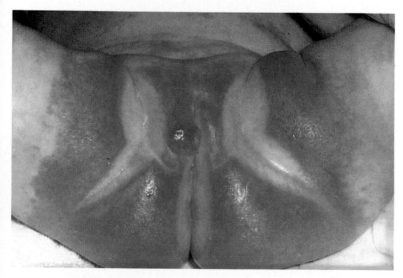

Fig. 31 Ammoniacal napkin rash.

5 | Atopic Eczema (1)

Asthma, hay fever and infantile eczema tend to run in families. Up to 25% of the population are potentially 'atopic' although less than 10% develop eczema.

Synonym
Infantile eczema.

Aetiology
Inheritance of atopic diathesis. Sensitivity/allergy to foreign proteins (type I hypersensitivity reactions). A generally intolerant and vulnerable ('leaky') skin. Eczema made worse by cold (low humidity), heat, woollen clothing, infections and stress.

Clinical features
Atopic eczema can occur at any age, but often develops about 3 months after birth. Intense pruritus is a prominent feature (Fig. 32)

Facial
The face is often involved in babies (Fig. 33). Itchy, erythematous papules on the cheeks or erythematosquamous dry/'chapped' or hypopigmented areas may be seen. Infraorbital lines (Morgan's folds) are common in atopic individuals.

Flexural
Characteristic in early childhood. Symmetrical involvement of elbow and knee flexures, wrists and ankles. The skin is generally dry and lichenified or excoriated. Constant licking of lips in some children causes 'lick eczema' (Fig. 34).

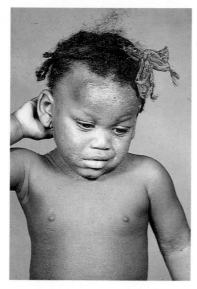 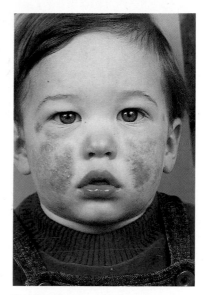

Fig. 32 Childhood atopic eczema.   **Fig. 33** facial atopic eczema.

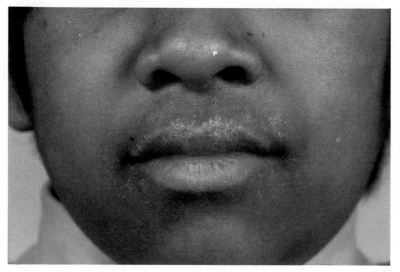

Fig. 34 'Lick eczema'.

5 | Atopic Eczema (2)

Reverse pattern
The extensor surfaces of arms and legs are involved in some children. The pattern of eczema in these cases is frequently 'discoid' (Fig. 35). A 'papular' form of eczema is common in Negroes. (Fig. 36)

Lichenification
Constant rubbing and scratching gives rise to areas of thickened skin with increased skin markings. This is particularly seen around flexures (Fig. 37).

Secondary infection
This is common and may both exacerbate eczema and produce local lymphadenopathy (Fig. 39).

Eczema herpeticum
Herpes simplex (and in the past vaccinia) may disseminate widely in patients with atopic eczema (Fig. 40). Viral warts and molluscum contagiosum also occur more commonly in atopics.

Superficial, hypopigmented
Patches of eczema affecting the face in children (Fig. 38) (*pityriasis alba*) and *forefoot eczema* (*juvenile plantar dermatosis*) (Fig. 41) may occur in both atopic and non-atopic children. Their isolated occurrence does not necessarily confirm atopy. Chapping and frictional factors are usually important.

'Nappy rash'
Primary irritant napkin dermatitis may occasionally be the first manifestation of atopic eczema (see also p. 19).

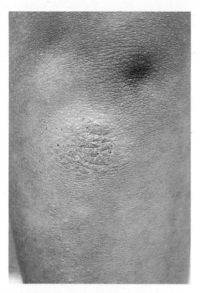

Fig. 35 Extensor discoid atopic eczema with post-inflammatory hypopigmentation.

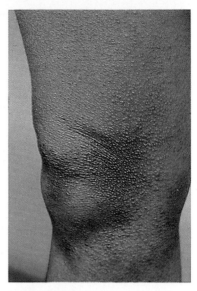

Fig. 36 Follicular/papular eczema.

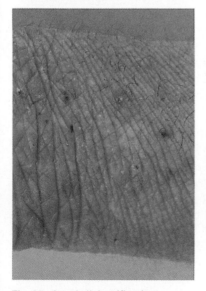

Fig. 37 Atopic lichenification.

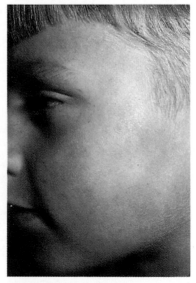

Fig. 38 Pityriasis alba (chronic superficial depigmenting dermatitis).

Atopic Eczema (3)

Treatment

Soap substitutes and water softeners/bath emollients, e.g. emulsifying ointment, oatmeal preparations, bath oils, should be used.

Emollients, e.g. E45 cream, oily cream and simple ointment need to be used frequently to help hydrate the skin.

Tar preparations, e.g. coal tar paste or coal tar paste bandages are useful in chronic or lichenified eczema (applied on top of steroid).

Topical steroids are extremely effective. The potency of steroids used will depend on age, extent and activity of eczema. In general, hydrocortisone is preferred for children and facial/flexural skin but short bursts of stronger steroids may be required to bring eczema under control.

Topical antibiotics may be required for infected eczema; these are often combined with a topical steroid. Systemic antibiotics are also often necessary.

Sedative antihistamines help to reduce pruritus, especially at night.

Wool causes itching. Cotton clothing is preferable.

Wet compresses are very helpful in the initial management of acute eczema.

Eczema herpeticum is a medical emergency and systemic Acyclovir will normally be required.

Counselling about the possible role of house dust mite, dietary factors, etc. should be given to parents, and children should be given career advice so as to avoid irritant and wet work.

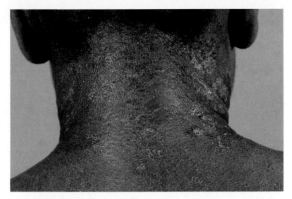

Fig. 39 Secondarily infected atopic eczema.

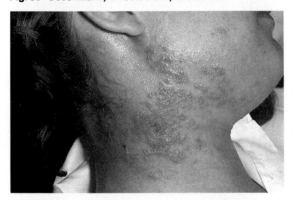

Fig. 40 Extensive herpes simplex in an atopic.

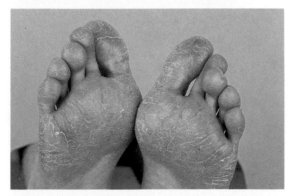

Fig. 41 Juvenile plantar dermatosis. The result of friction and occlusive footwear.

Tinea/pityriasis amiantacea

Aetiology

Distinctive reaction pattern of scalp. May be associated with psoriasis/eczema.

Clinical features

Asbestos-like, silvery scales adhere firmly to scalp and hair (Fig. 42). If there is associated infection the underlying scalp is erythematous and moist. There may be some loss of hair.

Treatment

1–5% salicylic acid in arachis oil, tar shampoo, steroid/antibacterial cream. Occasionally systemic antibiotics and stronger tar preparations.

Cradle cap (seborrhoeic eczema)

Aetiology

Unknown. Possible constitutional and microbial factors.

Clinical features

Appears at 0–3 months. The scalp is covered with 'greasy' scales (Fig. 43). The cheeks, flexures of neck, axillae, napkin areas and ears are often affected. May mimic psoriasis.

Treatment

Mild keratolytics, e.g. 2% salicylic acid in arachis oil for the scalp; non-soap cleansers and hydrocortisone-antiseptic combinations elsewhere.

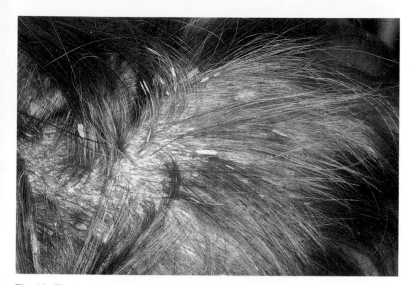

Fig. 42 Tinea amiantacea.

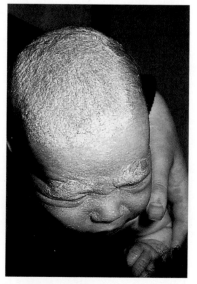

Fig. 43 Cradle cap.

Ringworm

Synonym

Tinea capitis.

Aetiology

Microsporum audouinii and *M. canis* invade hair shafts. The former condition is now, fortunately, a rarity. *M. canis* is, however, commonly contracted from cats and dogs (especially puppies). Animal trichophyton infections cause more severe reactions.

Clinical features

The condition is usually seen in children and produces circular, erythematous bald patches with scaling and broken hair shafts (Fig. 44). Wood's light examination shows a green/blue fluorescence for *M. audouinii* or *M. canis* (Fig. 45) but not for other types of fungus. A more inflammatory reaction follows infection with animal ringworm (cows, horses, etc.) (Fig. 46). This produces a tender and much more pustular *kerion* (Fig. 47). This may ultimately cause scarring alopecia. Fungal microscopy and culture is usually positive, but false-negative results may occur with kerion.

Treatment

Oral griseofulvin is the treatment of choice. The affected hair should be 'cropped' short and treatment continued for at least 6 weeks. Topical antifungal agents may also be used.

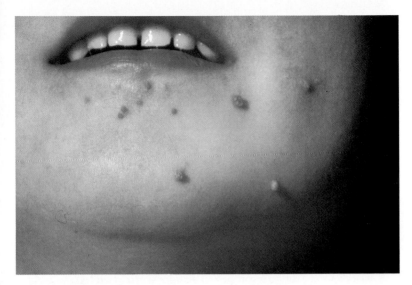

Fig. 51 Filiform warts.

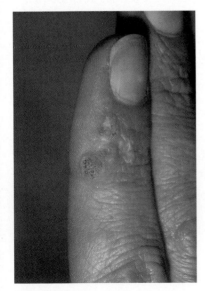

Fig. 52 Common warts.

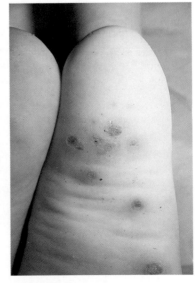

Fig. 53 Multiple plantar warts.

Warts (cont)

Plantar warts (verrucae)

Clinical features

Deep, hyperkeratotic, often tender lesions on the sole (Fig. 53). Body weight causes them to grow inwards rather than outwards. Differentiated from corns/calluses by paring; warts have areas of black speckling and fine bleeding points. Multiple superficial plantar warts may coalesce to form a 'mosaic wart' which is very resistant to therapy and implies poor natural resistance (Fig. 54).

Treatment

Combination of paring and salicylic acid plasters or paints (under occlusion). Weekly applications of monochloracetic acid (caution: highly caustic) or intermittent treatment with liquid NO_2. Therapy may be required for several weeks or months. Curettage and cautery may be employed for the occasional resistant verruca but is painful even with local anaesthetic.

Plane warts (Fig. 55)

Clinical features

Occur in young children, occasionally in adults. Multiple smooth, small, flat-topped papules which may be linear or coalesce due to trauma (Koebner phenomenon) (Fig. 56). The face and backs of hands are particularly affected. They persist longer than other warts and respond less well to treatment. They will eventually disappear spontaneously.

Treatment

2% salicylic acid in 70% spirit lotion is usually adequate (as placebo).

Genital warts (condyloma acuminata)

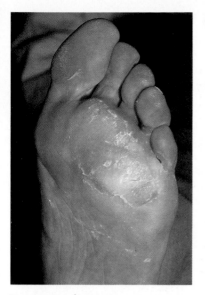

Fig. 54 Mosaic plantar wart.

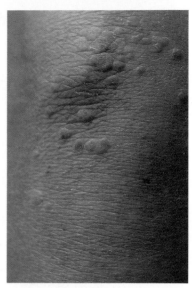

Fig. 55 Plane warts.

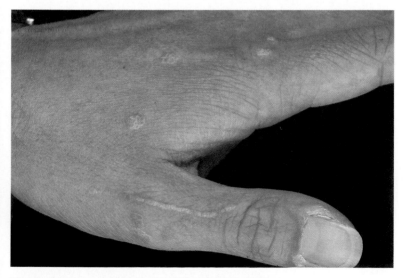

Fig. 56 Plane warts showing Koebner phenomenon.

Molluscum contagiosum (Fig. 57)

Aetiology

Pox virus.

Clinical features

Common in childhood, especially in atopics. Lesions are characteristically grouped, pearly white or pink, firm, umbilicated papules with a central depression and commonly affect the face, neck, trunk and perineum although any area may be involved. They may grow to 5–10 mm in diameter if left untreated, and soften as they mature. Some become inflamed or 2° infected.

Treatment

Lesions are easily removed with a sharp wooden cocktail stick or may be 'spiked' with phenol or iodine or painted with podophyllin. They can also be removed by curettage, cryotherapy, diathermy or any other mildly traumatic procedure.

Hand, foot and mouth disease

Aetiology

A Coxsackie infection. Epidemic. Mainly affecting young children.

Clinical features

The disease is usually mild, with an incubation period of 5–7 days. There are scattered vesicles in the mouth and on the palms/soles (Fig. 58). Those in the mouth soon break down to leave small ulcers (Fig. 59). In some children there may be a more widespread exanthem.

Treatment

None.

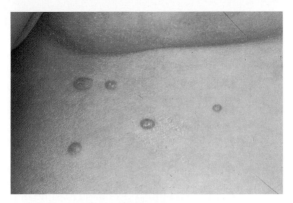

Fig. 57 Molluscum contagiosum.

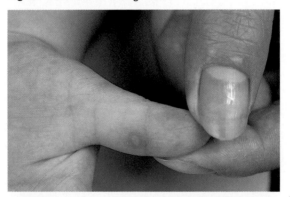

Fig. 58 Characteristic vesicle in hand, foot and mouth disease.

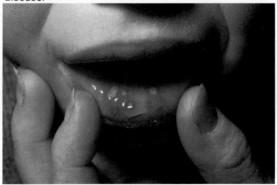

Fig. 59 Oral involvement in hand, foot and mouth disease.

9 | Childhood Infestations

Head lice (pediculosis capitis)

Aetiology

Common infestation (Fig. 60) in unhygienic or crowded conditions.

Clinical features

Severe pruritus, especially on the nape of neck and occiput. Lice may be present but nits (eggs) on hair shafts are diagnostic. Excoriations are common. Impetiginous secondary infection can occur. Exudation may cause matting of hair.

Treatment

Removal of nits with a fine-toothed metal comb. 0.5% malathion or 0.5% carbaryl solution applied to hair after washing. Repeated treatments may be necessary. Contacts must also be treated.

Insect bites (papular urticaria; heat bumps) (Fig. 61)

Aetiology

Hypersensitivity reaction to insect bites, e.g. fleas, bedbugs, mites.

Clinical features

Urticated papules occur in groups (Fig. 62) and may be seasonal. Bullae can occur, particularly on the legs. Pruritus may be intense. Episodes may be recurrent or persist for several months. Impetigo can be a complication.

Treatment

Symptomatic. Treat source if possible (including pets). Systemic antihistamines and topical steroids may be useful.

See also Scabies (p. 95).

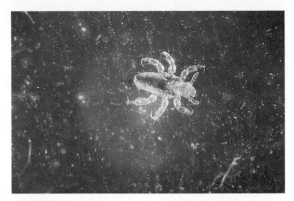

Fig. 60 Head louse.

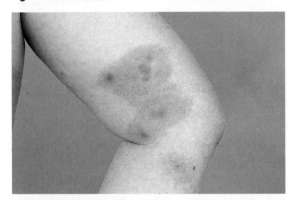

Fig. 61 Papular urticaria (bites).

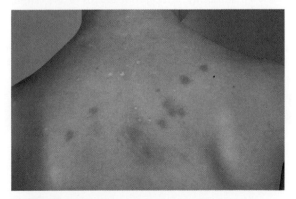

Fig. 62 Characteristic pattern of lesions as seen in insect bites.

10 | Childhood Reactions

Henoch-Schönlein purpura (allergic vasculitis)

Aetiology

An immune complex hypersensitivity reaction to streptococcal infection.

Clinical features

Palpable (papular) purpura affects the lower legs, thighs and buttocks (Fig. 63); sometimes urticarial or necrotic. There may be arthralgia, abdominal pain, vomiting and bloody diarrhoea; renal damage may lead to proliferative glomerulonephritis with nephritis or nephrotic syndromes. ESR and ASO titres may be raised. The urine should be checked regularly for protein, casts and haematuria.

Treatment

Bed-rest in the acute stage. Penicillin for streptococcal infections; sometimes systemic steroids. Prognosis is generally good but depends on renal involvement.

Acute urticaria (hives; nettle rash)

Aetiology

Mast cell degranulation with histamine release due to drugs, foods, infections or infestations.

Clinical features

Increased incidence in atopics. Itchy weals arise suddenly, within minutes or hours (Figs. 64, 65). There may be associated angioedema and eosinophilia.

Treatment

Treat any underlying infestation or infection. Try elimination diets. Antihistamines. Avoid aspirin.

DERMATOLOGY

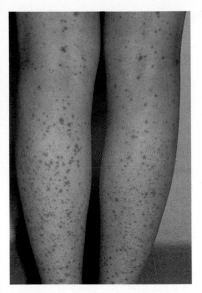

Fig. 63 Henoch-Schönlein type purpura.

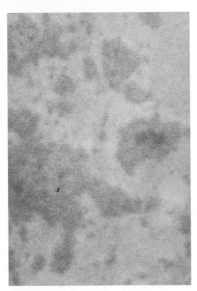

Fig. 64 Urticarial weals.

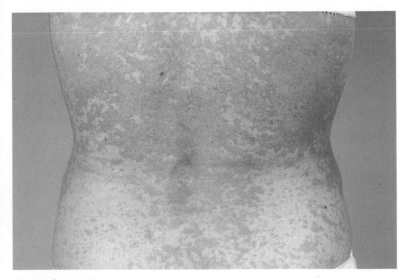

Fig. 65 Generalised urticaria.

11 | Acne Vulgaris (1)

Acne is an inflammatory disorder of the pilosebaceous follicles which occurs particularly at adolescence when sebaceous glands become active.

Aetiology

Several factors are of importance:
1. Genetic
2. Androgenic (and, to some degree, progesterogenic) stimulation
3. Abnormal sebum production
4. Colonisation of pilosebaceous unit with proprioni bacterium acnes
5. Obstruction of the sebaceous duct
6. Inflammation.

Clinical features

The characteristic lesion is the *comedone* (Fig. 66) which presents as a dark, follicular plug (blackhead), or a small papule (closed comedone). Secondary inflammation causes papules and pustules which may affect the face, chest, back and shoulders (Fig. 67). Pre-menstrual flares are common in women. Deeper *nodulocystic acne* produces severe scarring (Fig. 68) and occurs more commonly in men, as does *acne conglobata* (Fig. 69), an uncommon, severe, recalcitrant form of acne. There are multiple 'paired' comedones with connecting sinuses, on the back, chest, neck and face. Large (conglobate) cysts may develop and there is often scarring or acne-keloid formation (Figs. 70, 71).

DERMATOLOGY

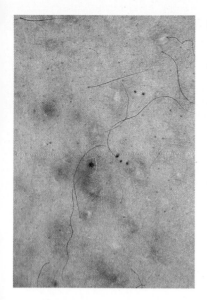

Fig. 66 Paired comedones as seen in acne conglobata.

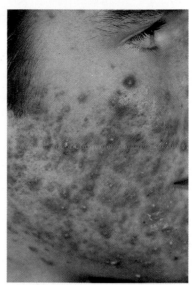

Fig. 67 Superficial inflammatory acne.

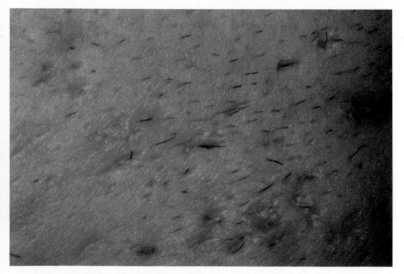

Fig. 68 Post acne ('ice-pick') scarring.

Management

Topical therapy
Keratolytics are beneficial for superficial inflammatory acne. *Benzoyl peroxide* has both an antibacterial and a drying/peeling action. *Retinoic acid* is useful for comedonal acne although it may have an irritant effect and intermittent use of the cream formulation is recommended initially. *Topical antibiotics* such as 1.5% clindamycin with 10% propylene glycol in 70% spirit lotion or one of the newer topical tetracyclines (Topicycline) help. *Ultraviolet B light* and *natural sunlight* are often beneficial and produce erythema and slight peeling. Intralesional half-strength steroid is sometimes useful for inflammatory nodulocystic lesions.

Systemic therapy
Oral antibiotics—oxytetracycline or erythromycin 500 mg b.d. produce improvement in about 70% of patients. For tetracycline, it is important that *therapy* is taken with water and away from food. For maintenance therapy, antibiotics may be given at lower dose but they will need to be continued for some months/years. *Oral contraceptives* containing high (50 μg) levels of oestrogen doses, such as Diane, may be helpful. *Oral retinoids* (13 cis retinoic acid) can produce a dramatic improvement in severe nodulocystic acne. Teratogenic side-effects limit its use in women and the treatment is at present only available in hospital.

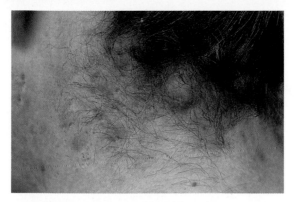

Fig. 69 Acne conglobata of neck.

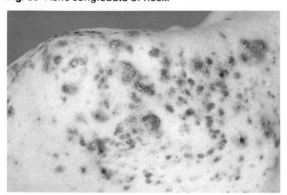

Fig. 70 Severe nodulocystic acne.

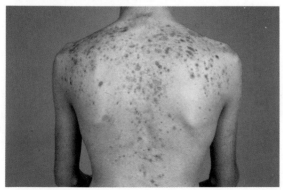

Fig. 71 Post-acne scarring.

Aetiology

Psoriasis affects approximately 2% of the population. Genetic factors are important; 40% of patients have a positive family history. Rapid epidermal transit time with increased epidermal cell production.

Clinical features

Plaque psoriasis characterised by well-demarcated, erythematous areas covered with thick, silvery scales (Fig. 72). Pinpoint capillary bleeding when scales are removed. Symmetrical plaques commonly affect extensor surfaces, especially the elbows and knees. Frequently affects scalp and sacrum (Fig. 74), but patches may occur anywhere on the body. May develop at site of trauma (Koebner phenomenon) (Fig. 73).
Guttate (and exanthematic) psoriasis (Figs. 75, 76, 77) commoner in the young and often precipitated by a streptococcal sore throat. Multiple 'rain-drop' lesions occur suddenly on trunk and limbs. The condition may resolve spontaneously or individual spots may enlarge and turn to plaque psoriasis.
Pustular psoriasis (Fig. 78).   Rare generalised form which can be fatal. Patients are often erythrodermic with sheets of sterile pustules and associated fever, malaise and leukocytosis.
Flexural psoriasis (Fig. 79).   Loses its characteristic silvery scale but the well-demarcated erythematous areas remain and may mimic intertrigo, candidiasis and tinea.

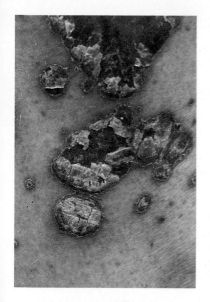

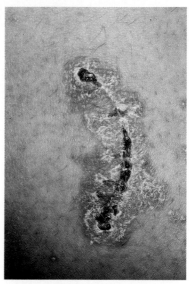

Fig. 72 Typical psoriatic plaques with thick silvery scales.

Fig. 73 Psoriasis showing Koebner phenomenon.

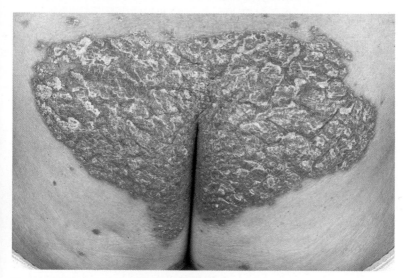

Fig. 74 Typical psoriatic plaque on sacrum.

Erythrodermic psoriasis. When psoriasis involves the whole body the resulting erythroderma may be difficult to differentiate from other types of erythrodermic exfoliative dermatoses (Fig. 80). Such patients lose their ability to control body temperature and fluid balance, and risk both infection and cardiac and renal failure.

Persistent palmoplantar pustulosis (Fig. 81). Often regarded as a localised form of psoriasis of the hands and feet, but frequently occurs without evidence of psoriasis elsewhere. Localised patches of erythema and scaling occur on the palms and soles with scattered, sterile, yellow-brown pustules. The condition is very resistant to treatment.

Scalp psoriasis. Multiple discrete plaques or involvement of entire scalp and/or ears and scalp margins. Plaques are frequently thick, particularly at the occiput, but alopecia is uncommon (p. 153).

Nail psoriasis. Commonly affected by several abnormalities—pitting, onycholysis, subungual hyperkeratosis, salmon patch (p. 149).

Psoriatic arthropathy. Commonly affects the terminal interphalangeal joints and sacroiliac joints, but both large and small joints may be involved. A severe destructive form of arthritis known as 'arthritis mutilans' is occasionally seen.

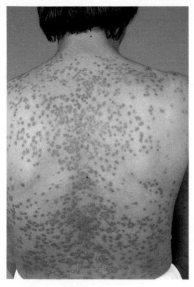

Fig. 75 Guttate psoriasis.

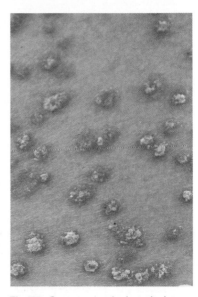

Fig. 76 Guttate psoriasis: raindrop lesions.

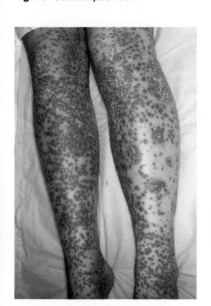

Fig. 77 Exanthematic psoriasis.

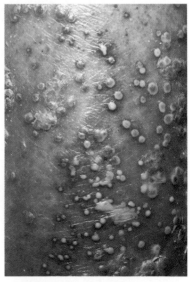

Fig. 78 Pustular psoriasis.

Treatment

Topical steroids. Effective, but continued use may lead to lessening of effect and some destabilisation of ordinary plaque psoriasis. Better employed (in a descending sequence of potency) in combination with another treatment modality, e.g. tar. This combines the rapid initial benefits and cosmetic acceptability of topical steroids (by day) with the slower but more long-lasting effects of a coal tar preparation (at night). Weaker steroid or steroid/antiseptic preparations remain very useful for intertriginous areas.

Tar. Either alone or combined with salicylic acid. Cleaner forms now available.

Ultravoilet light (UVB). E_0-E_1 dose alone or combined with tar/tar baths. Newer treatment combining psoralen with UVA (PUVA) is even more successful at clearing extensive refractory psoriasis.

Dithranol. Useful for plaque psoriasis in in-patients. Diluted in Lassar's Paste, initially at 0.1%. Cleaner forms now available for out-patient used to be used at normal concentrations overnight or in high concentrations for just half-an-hour. May be combined with tar baths and UVB.

Systemic therapy. Cystotoxic drugs, e.g. methotrexate, etretinate, etc. are treatments normally only initiated by dermatologists.

Scalp psoriasis. Keratolytics, tar shampoos, topical steroids as lotions/gels.

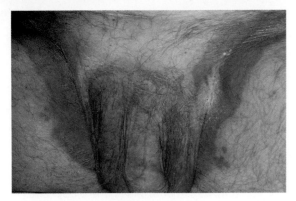

Fig. 79 Flexural psoriasis.

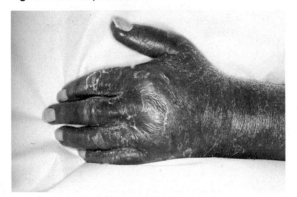

Fig. 80 Exfoliative/erythrodermic psoriasis.

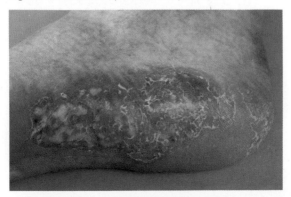

Fig. 81 Persistent palmoplantar pustulosis.

Lichen simplex (neurodermatitis)

Aetiology

A localised, sometimes eczematous response to constant rubbing; often partly habit and frequently triggered by stress.

Clinical features

Several characteristic patterns: in women, the nape of neck, side of neck, vulva; in men, the ankle/shin (Fig. 82), scrotum and perianal area (Fig. 83); in both sexes, the elbow and central palms. Usually solitary, well-demarcated, lichenified lesions, more diffuse on scrotum and perianal area, due to repeated scratching and rubbing (Fig. 84).

Treatment

Potent topical steroids, tar or tar paste bandages, sedative antihistamines, occasionally intralesional steroids.

Pruritus ani (Fig. 85)

Aetiology

Pre-disposing factors include haemorrhoids, fissures, irritation from mucous or faecal leak, sweat/maceration, contact dermatitis, threadworm infection (in children).

Clinical features

Lichen simplex, maceration, fissuring or bacterial/candidal intertrigo.

Treatment

Treat underlying or complicating factors. Soap substitutes, mild/moderate corticosteroid/antiseptic preparations. Sedative antihistamines.

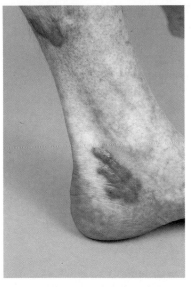

Fig. 82 Lichen simplex chronicus.

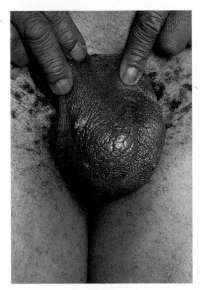

Fig. 83 Lichen simplex of scrotum.

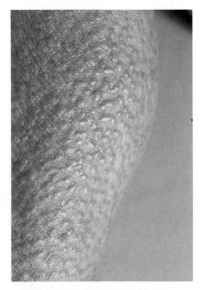

Fig. 84 Pebbly lichenification from constant rubbing.

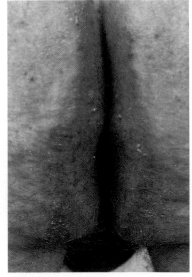

Fig. 85 Pruritus ani/perianal dermatitis.

Prurigo

Clinical features

'Prurigo' is a term used to describe any localised skin abnormality where the principal symptom is itch. Lesions include excoriations, prurigo nodules and localised areas of lichen simplex.
'Cape prurigo'. A common pattern in the elderly (Fig. 86). Dry skin and low serum iron are important factors.
'Tycoon scalp'. A characteristic pattern of excoriation of the scalp, mainly affecting businessmen and frequently associated with stress. Folliculitis and seborrhoeic dermatitis may be initiating factors (Fig. 87).
Subacute prurigo. Mainly affects the extensor aspects of limbs in women but more diffuse patterns also occur.
Nodular prurigo. An intransigent pattern of prurigo with intensely pruriginous nodules separated by areas of normal skin. Mainly affects the extensor aspects of limbs (Fig. 88).

Treatment

'Cape' prurigo often responds to simple emollients, iron replacement therapy and sedative antihistamines. Crotamiton/hydrocortisone cream is also helpful. Other patterns of prurigo are very intransigent and respond poorly to treatment. The itch/scratch/itch habit is difficult to break. Potent steroids, occlusive tar paste bandages, sedative antihistamines and, occasionally, intralesional steroids are required.

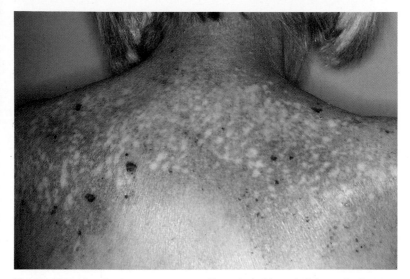

Fig. 86 'Cape prurigo': a common manifestation of iron deficiency in the elderly.

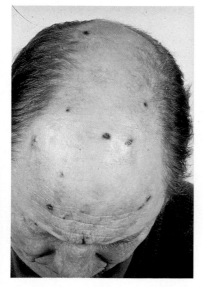

Fig. 87 Tycoon scalp.

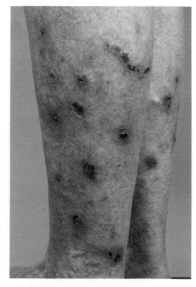

Fig. 88 Nodular prurigo.

14 | Lichen Planus

Aetiology

The cause is unknown, although an autoimmune basis has been suggested.

Clinical features

The characteristic skin lesions are small, itchy, shiny, flat-topped, violaceous papules (Fig. 89) with an overlying network of fine white lines (Wickham's striae) (Fig. 90). The eruption usually affects the wrists, forearms and trunk, lasting from 6 months to 2 years. The mouth (and genitalia) are also often affected with typical milky, 'lace-like' streaks or violaceous/atrophic patches. Scalp involvement may produce scarring alopecia, and permanent nail loss may occur if nail involvement is severe. Lesions occurring on the shins tend to coalesce and produce hypertrophic plaques (Fig. 91). Fading skin papules leave post-inflammatory hyperpigmentation. Lichen planus may also occur at sites of trauma (Fig. 92). This is known as the 'Koebner phenomenon' and is also seen in psoriasis and with certain viral infections such as molluscum contagiosum and plane warts.

Treatment

Topical steroids and sedative antihistamines are helpful for symptomatic relief, although in mild cases no treatment may be required. Hypertrophic plaques can be treated with potent topical steroids or injected with intralesional steroids. There are also several proprietary steroid and anti-inflammatory agents that can be used for the mouth.

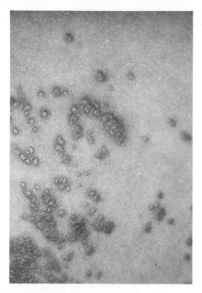

Fig. 89 Flat-topped violaceous papules of lichen planus.

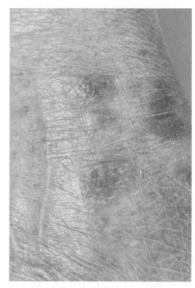

Fig. 90 Wickham's striae (lichen planus).

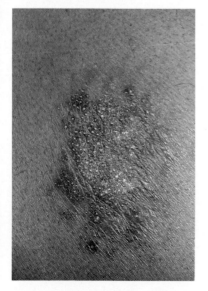

Fig. 91 Hypertrophic lichen planus.

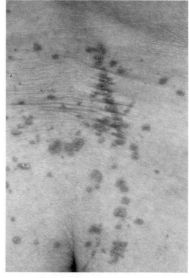

Fig. 92 Lichen planus (Koebner phenomenon).

15 | Pityriasis Rosea

Pityriasis rosea is a common, self-limiting eruption which predominantly affects young adults.

Aetiology

The cause is unknown; an infective agent has been suggested but not isolated.

Clinical features

Characteristically, the initial lesion is a solitary oval, erythematous, scaly 'herald patch', often on the trunk (Fig. 93). Similar, but smaller lesions appear after an interval of 1 or 2 weeks over the trunk, neck and upper arms in a symmetrical and generalised distribution. Individual lesions lie parallel to the ribs, creating a 'Christmas tree' pattern (Fig. 94). Pruritus is minimal, but occasionally there may be malaise and lymphadenopathy. The eruption usually fades within 4–6 weeks.

Management

Usually no treatment is required. Mild topical steroids may hasten resolution or help the more 'eczematous' cases.

DERMATOLOGY

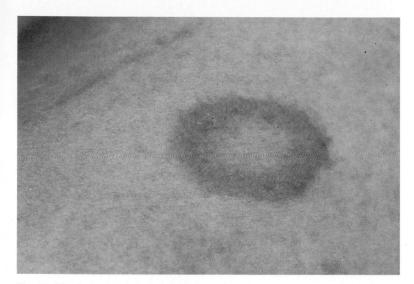

Fig. 93 Pityriasis rosea: 'herald patch'.

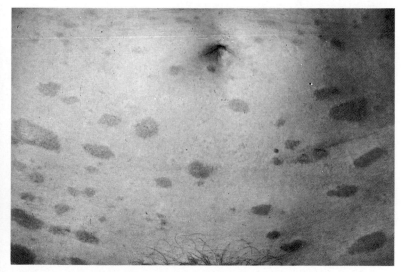

Fig. 94 Typical distribution of lesions in pityriasis rosea.

16 | Pityriasis Lichenoides

Aetiology

Unknown.

Clinical features

Two forms exist.
Acute. Adolescents are usually affected. Small, red papules occur on the trunk and limbs. The lesions become vesicular and then necrotic and ulcerate to produce pitted scars. Fever and systemic upset may occur. Mucous membranes may be involved. The eruption is often mistaken for chickenpox (Figs. 95, 96).
Chronic. Small, reddish or orange-brown papules occur. Some may become purpuric whilst others develop a characteristic 'mica' scale. Lesions resolve slowly, leaving either a brown hyperpigmented or hypopigmented area. There is no systemic upset. The condition may grumble on for months/years (Figs. 97, 98).

Treatment

None may be necessary.
Ultraviolet light (UVB), PUVA and sunshine are all useful in the chronic form. Tar baths may be combined with both sun and UVB.

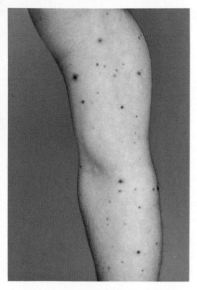

Fig. 95 Pityriasis lichenoides acuta.

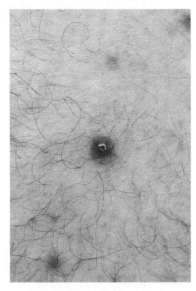

Fig. 96 Close-up of an early lesion of pityriasis lichenoides.

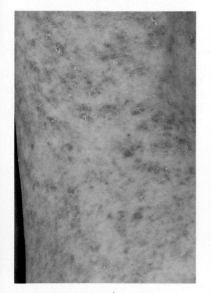

Fig. 97 Pityriasis lichenoides chronica.

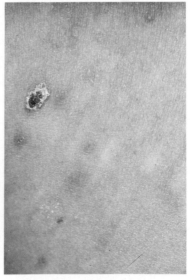

Fig. 98 Pityriasis lichenoides chronica with post-inflammatory hypopigmentation.

17 | Cutaneous Reaction Patterns (1)

Chronic urticaria (Fig. 99)

Aetiology

An increase in vascular permeability/reactivity. Both immune (type I and III) and non-immune (pharmacological) mechanisms may play a part. Histamine is the most common mediator. Frequent precipitating factors include:
1. Drugs, e.g. aspirin, penicillin
2. Food additives, e.g. tartrazine (E102)
3. Fungal/yeast infections, e.g. thrush
4. Parasites, e.g. intestinal worms
5. Other infections
6. Disorders of the immune system, e.g. SLE, complement deficiency
7. Stress.
In many cases no obvious cause is found.

Clinical features

Transient raised weals varying from a few mm to several cm in size (Fig. 100). Limbs and trunk are particularly affected but lesions may occur anywhere. Weals are extremely itchy, last from 4–24 hours and fade completely. Pressure sites are commonly affected and most patients are also dermographic (Fig. 101). There may be associated angioedema. Rarely, there is overlap with urticarial vasculitis.

Treatment

Avoid aspirin and any other drugs that may have been implicated. Treat any underlying bacterial, fungal or parasitic infection. Elimination diets (especially a dye and preservative-free diet) may help. Antihistamines give relief; severely affected patients may require systemic steroids.

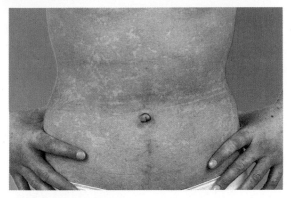

Fig. 99 Giant urticaria.

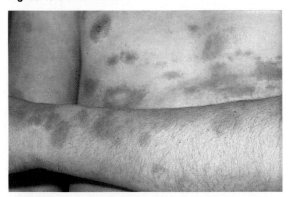

Fig. 100 Urticarial weals.

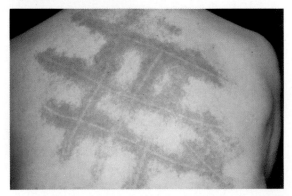

Fig. 101 Exaggerated weal and flare (dermographism).

17 | Cutaneous Reaction Patterns (2)

Angioedema

Aetiology

Hereditary angioedema is an autosomal dominant condition due to C1 esterase inhibitor deficiency in the complement cascade. Angioedema may also occur as part of the symptom complex in both acute and chronic urticaria.

Clinical features

Angioedema produces swelling of the lips (Figs. 102, 103), periorbital area (Fig. 104), neck and joints. The larynx may be affected and such involvement can be fatal. Gut involvement may produce abdominal pains. Urticaria is not normally a feature of true hereditary angioedema but the latter may occur in cases of ordinary urticaria.

Treatment

Anyone who suffers recurrent attacks of angioedema or in whom there is a family history of angioedema should be positively screened for C1 esterase inhibitor deficiency. Specific drugs such as stanozolol, tranexamic acid and danazol are the only effective prophylactic agents for hereditary angioedema. Acute episodes require injection of C1 esterase inhibitor or infusion of fresh frozen plasma. Angioedema associated with ordinary urticaria may be treated with antihistamines and/or steroids. Severe attacks should be treated as for anaphylaxis, with 0.5 ml 1/1 000 adrenalin by subcutaneous injection.

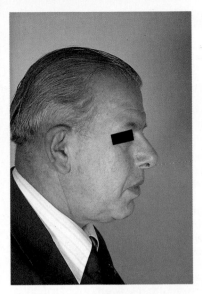

Fig. 102 Aspirin-induced angioedema (before).

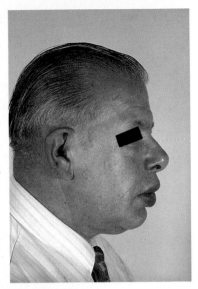

Fig. 103 Aspirin-induced angioedema (after).

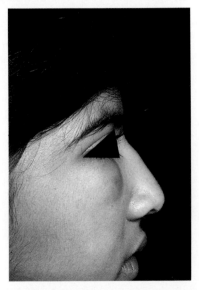

Fig. 104 Periorbital swelling (recurrent angioedema).

Erythema multiforme

Aetiology

A localised form of vasculitis. Attacks may be triggered by drugs and viral infections (especially herpes simplex and *Mycoplasma*).

Clinical features

The eruption can occur at any age. There may be a prodromal illness. Initial lesions are dull, red, flat maculopapules spreading centrifugally, the centre becoming cyanotic, purpuric or even bullous or necrotic (Fig. 105). The characteristic target or iris lesions (Fig. 106) symmetrically involve the periphery, e.g. palms, dorsae of hands, feet, knees, elbows and forearms. Mucous membranes may be affected. A severe bullous form of erythema multiforme, Stevens-Johnson syndrome, with particular involvement of mucous membranes, can occur (Fig. 107). There is associated pyrexia and malaise, with oral, ocular and genital lesions. This form carries a significant morbidity and mortality.

Treatment

Usually symptomatic. Steroids may reduce the severity of attacks. The underlying cause should be removed or treated, where possible. Patients with severe recurrent erythema multiforme caused by herpes simplex may require treatment with continuous prophylactic acyclovir or by regular bi-monthly injections of gamma-globulin.

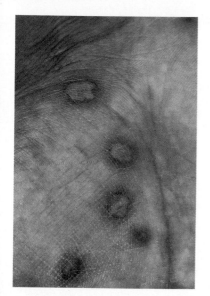

Fig. 105 Bullous erythema multiforme lesions of palm.

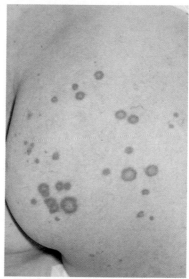

Fig. 106 Erythema multiforme: typical target or iris lesions.

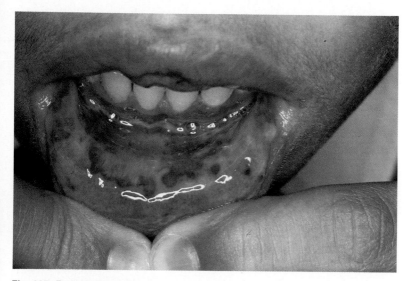

Fig. 107 Erythema multiforme: mucosal involvement.

Systemic Reaction Patterns (2)

Erythema nodosum

Aetiology

A common vasculitis reaction of larger subcutaneous vessels, due to a variety of provoking agents.

1. Sarcoidosis
2. Infections
   —Streptococcus
   —Tuberculosis
   —Infectious mononucleosis
   —Viral
   —Chlamydia
3. Drugs
   —Sulphonamides
   —Oral contraceptives
   —Salicylates
   —Bromides/iodides
   —Gold salts
4. Inflammatory bowel disease.

Clinical features

There may be a prodromal illness. Erythematous, tender, nodules appear on shins (Fig. 108) and occasionally thighs and forearms. There is associated pyrexia, malaise, oedema and aching of legs. The colour changes from bright red to purple to leave a brownish 'bruise'. Lesions occur in crops and recurrences may occur. Most attacks settle within 2–12 weeks.

Treatment

Bed-rest, anti-inflammatory analgesics and support stockings or bandages. Systemic steroids may be required for severe cases.

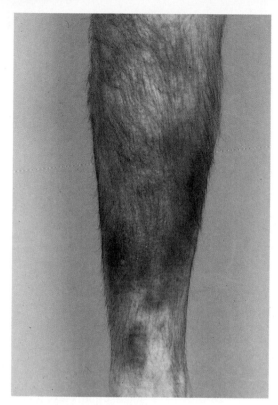

Fig. 108 Erythema nodosum.

Systemic Reaction Patterns (3)

Vasculitis (Fig. 109)

Aetiology

Immune complex deposition in blood vessels. Drugs, infections, ingested allergens and autoantigens have all been implicated.

Clinical features

Classically, the lower legs are affected. Urticaria, toxic erythema and palpable purpura may progress to necrotic or bullous lesions (Fig. 110) with crusting and ulceration. Possible associated systemic vasculitis with renal, gastrointestinal and respiratory involvement and arthritis.

Treatment

Investigation of the underlying cause. Bed-rest. Systemic steroids may be required.

Capillaritis

Aetiology

Capillary leakage/vasculitis (Fig. 111). Most causes are cryptogenic, e.g. Schamberg's capillaritis, but some drugs produce a similar eruption. Stasis factors are also important.

Clinical features

The idiopathic type usually affects the lower legs of young men. Discrete areas of asymptomatic red-brown, petechial or punctate purpura— become hyperpigmented.

Treatment

Support stockings may help.

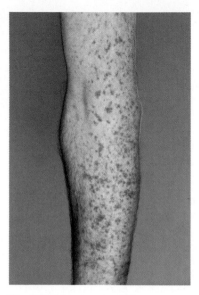

Fig. 109 Allergic vasculitis.

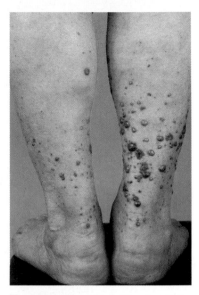

Fig. 110 Leukocytoclastic vasculitis.

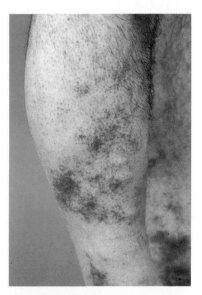

Fig. 111 Capillaritis with 'cayenne pepper' pigmentation.

19 | Rosacea

Aetiology

Unknown. Increased lability and reactivity of the facial vasculature.

Clinical features

Initially, transient flushing but later a persistent and diffuse facial erythema with inflamed papules and pustules (acne rosacea) and telangectasia. Chiefly involves glabella, cheeks, nose and chin. Lymphoedema, conjunctival suffusion, conjunctivitis, blepharitis and (rarely) keratitis. Exacerbation by sun, heat, alcohol, hot/spicy foods.
Rhinophyma. A variant seen mainly in men.

Treatment

Avoid precipitating factors. Oral oxytetracycline (papules and pustules) and oral clonidine (flushing). Rhinophyma usually requires plastic surgery. Low-dose antibiotics needed for months/years. Topical steroids are contraindicated.

Perioral dermatitis

Aetiology

Unknown. May develop from paraoral acne or paranasal seborrhoeic dermatitis. Prior use of a potent topical steroid is usually a factor.

Clinical features

Papulopustular eruption on a scaly, erythematous background around the mouth, nose and nasolabial folds. More frequent in women (Fig. 114).

Treatment

Systemic oxytetracycline (a reducing 4–6 week course), 1% hydrocortisone cream to reduce 'rebound' when potent steroids withdrawn.

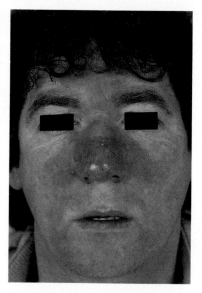

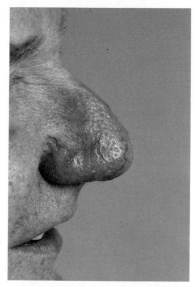

Fig. 112 Acne rosacea. Commoner in women, esp. those with Celtic skin. Cruciate distribution.

Fig. 113 Rhinophyma. Enlargement of the nose due to hypertrophy of sebaceous glands.

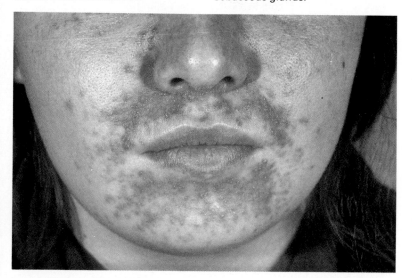

Fig. 114 Perioral dermatitis.

Dermographism (Fig. 115)

Clinical features

Light pressure produces a weal and flare formation with itching at the site of trauma within 5 min. May be associated with chronic urticaria; asymptomatic in around 5% of normal population.

Treatment

None may be required, or antihistamines.

Cholinergic urticaria

Clinical features

Common, predominantly affecting young adults and involving mainly trunk and limbs. Extremely itchy, micropapular, urticarial weals occur in response to exercise, emotion, or heat (Fig. 116).

Treatment

Antihistamines and anticholinergics may be helpful. Tends to resolve spontaneously.

Pressure urticaria (Fig. 117)

Clinical features

Rare. May be a component of ordinary chronic urticaria. Continued pressure produces painful swollen, indurated urticarial areas after several hours. May persist for 1–2 days.

Treatment

Cyproheptadine or other antihistamines can be tried but response is often disappointing. Oral steroids may be required.

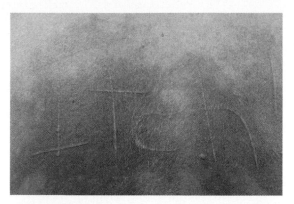

Fig. 115 Dermographism.

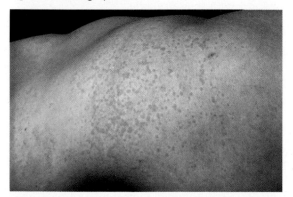

Fig. 116 Cholinergic urticaria.

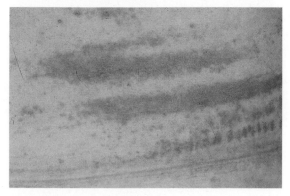

Fig. 117 Pressure urticaria.

Polymorphic light eruption (PMLE)
(Fig. 118)

Clinical features

Relatively common; usually affects young women, although it may occur at any age. Itchy papules or papulovesicles, erythema and urticated plaques develop within hours, mainly at sites recently exposed to sun. Starts in spring/early summer and declines thereafter. Tends to recur over many years. Sometimes associated with solar urticaria.

Treatment

Clothing and high protection sunscreens. Topical steroids and oral antihistamines. Tolerance can be induced. PUVA therapy can be given prophylactically to those severely affected. Mepacrine sometimes required for severe cases.

Hutchinson's summer prurigo
(Fig. 119)

Clinical features

Affects young children. There may be a family history. Itchy, erythematous, often excoriated papules on cheeks, nose and dorsum of hands.

Treatment

Symptomatic. Sunscreens partially helpful.

Juvenile spring eruption

Clinical features

Uncommon condition seen in boys more than girls. Erythema and pruritus of the ears is followed by grouped papules and vesicles. No treatment.

DERMATOLOGY

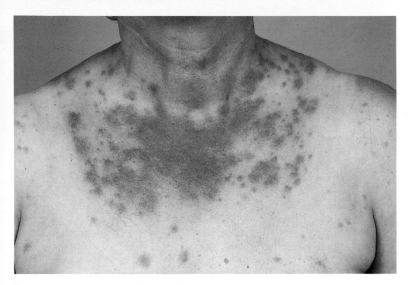

Fig. 118 Polymorphic light eruption.

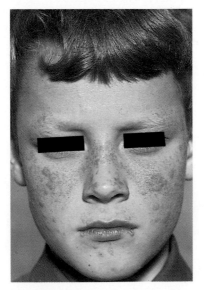

Fig. 119 Hutchinson's summer prurigo.

Photosensitive eczema/actinic reticuloid

Aetiology

1. Secondary to some eczemas—childhood atopic; seborrhoeic dermatitis in older men; volatile contact dermatitis, e.g. to Compositae.
2. Topically applied chemicals—tar, creosote.
3. Systemic drugs—thiazides, phenothiazines.

Clinical features

Mainly summer. Sensitivity is usually confined to short-wave UVL (UVB)/exposed areas but in actinic reticuloid may extend to include visible light, be year-long and generalised. Drug-induced photosensitivity is normally due to long-wave UVL (UVA) (Figs. 120, 121).

Treatment

Elimination of drug/easily avoided environmental causes. In constitutional eczema or those sensitised to a ubiquitous allergen, symptomatic treatment with topical steroids and broad spectrum sunscreens. In severe cases, systemic steroids and azathioprine.

Solar urticaria

Aetiology

Unknown. Abnormal reactivity to UVL.

Clinical features

Rare. Development of severely pruritic, erythematous weals within a few minutes of sun exposure. Resolve within about 1 h of sun avoidance. Erythropoietic protoporphyria must be excluded.

Treatment

Sun avoidance. Antihistamines no help.

DERMATOLOGY

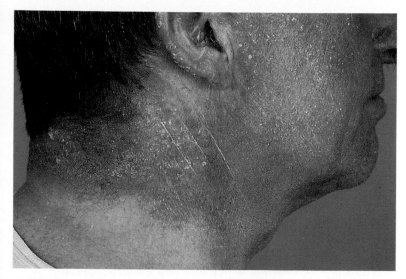

Fig. 120 Photodermatitis/relative sparing behind ear.

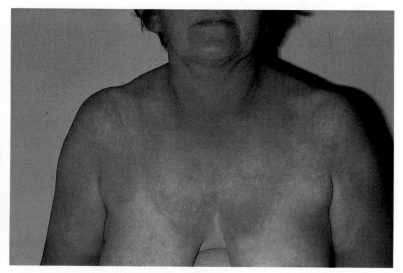

Fig. 121 Drug-induced photosensitivity.

Discoid lupus erythematosus (Fig. 122)

Aetiology

Autoimmune disorder.

Clinical features

Symmetrical, well-defined plaques of erythema with scaling, atrophy and follicular plugging. Mainly affecting light-exposed areas such as face, neck, scalp, ears, upper chest, back and backs of hands (Figs. 123, 124); frequently exacerbated by sunlight. Scalp involvement may produce scarring alopecia (Fig. 125). Rarely, there may also be associated systemic symptoms of lupus erythematosus.

Treatment

Avoidance of sunlight; sunscreens and topical steroids are helpful. Mepacrine or systemic steroids may be required.

Skin disorders usually aggravated by sunlight

Polymorphic light eruption and other photodermatoses; lupus erythematosus; porphyrias; rosacea; herpes simplex; erythema multiforme; benign lymphocytic infiltrations.

Skin disorders usually helped by sunlight

Psoriasis; acne vulgaris; pityriasis lichenoides; 'parapsoriasis'; mycosis fungoides.

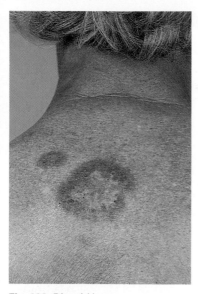

Fig. 122 Discoid lupus erythematosis.

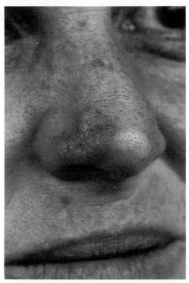

Fig. 123 Well-defined plaque of DLE on nose with follicular plugging/scarring.

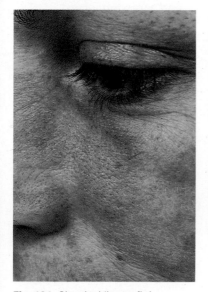

Fig. 124 Classical 'butterfly' distribution of DLE.

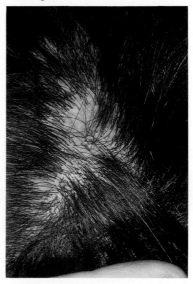

Fig. 125 Scarring alopecia.

The wide availability and use of drugs makes a drug history extremely important.

Aetiology

Hypersensitivity reactions can occur where the drug or drug metabolite acts as an antigen. Many eruptions remain, however, idiosyncratic.

Clinical features

Urticarial (p. 41), eczematous, bullous and lichenoid reactions may be seen. Specific eruption patterns include the following.

Morbilliform. Common maculopapular pattern of drug eruption which mimics viral exanthems. A good example of this is the ampicillin rash in patients with glandular fever. Other antibiotics and phenothiazines may give a similar reaction pattern (Fig. 126).

Purpuric (Fig. 129). Drugs can produce purpura by direct capillary damage or via thrombocytopenia, e.g. gold salts, quinine, quinidine, thiazides and benzodiazepines.

Vasculitis (p. 71) (Fig. 127). Produced by many drugs, including sulphonamides.

Erythema multiforme/Stevens-Johnson syndrome. Typical target lesions may be caused by barbiturates, phenytoin, gold, phenylbutazone and sulphonamides. Severe cases can progress to Stevens-Johnson syndrome with severe mucosal involvement (Fig. 128).

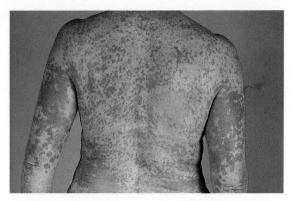

Fig. 126 Morbilliform 'ampicillin'-type rash.

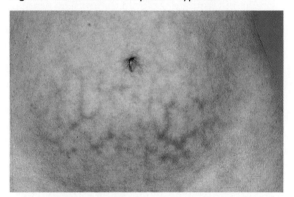

Fig. 127 Livedo vasculitis.

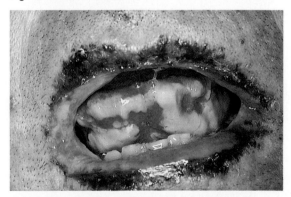

Fig. 128 Severe mucosal involvement in Stevens-Johnson syndrome.

Toxic epidermal necrolysis (p. 31). Large areas of epidermis are lost, leaving extensive, denuded areas of skin. Fluid loss, electrolyte imbalance and secondary infection are frequent complications. The condition has a significant mortality and may be caused by barbiturates, sulphonamides, hydantoin and phenylbutazone.

Fixed drug eruption (Fig. 130). These lesions are characerically well demarcated and dusky red, often with central blistering and subsequent post-inflammatory pigmentation. The eruption occurs at the same sites each time the responsible drug is taken. Laxatives containing phenol-phthalein, barbiturates and sulphonamides are common offenders.

Photosensitivity (p. 77). Phototoxic reactions can occur with drugs which would not usually produce a skin eruption without sun exposure. The distribution is typical, being confined to exposed areas, e.g. face, arms, 'V' of neck. Shaded areas such as those under the chin and ears are often spared.

Photoallergic reactions can also occur. Thiazides, sulphonamides, chlorpromazine, tetracyclines and nalidixic acid may all be responsible (Figs. 131, 132).

Treatment

Withdrawal of offending drug. Systemic steroids occasionally.

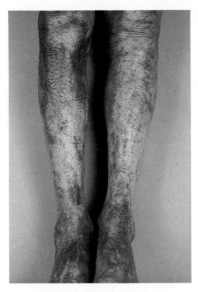

Fig. 129 Purpuric drug rash.

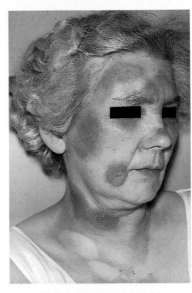

Fig. 130 Fixed drug eruption due to barbiturates, sulphonamides, etc.

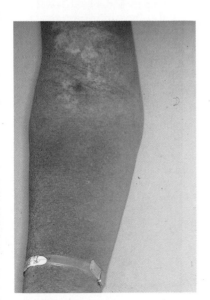

Fig. 131 Drug-induced erythroderma with islands of normal skin.

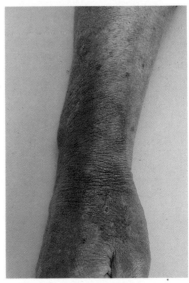

Fig. 132 Amiodarone pigmentation.

Bullous Disorders (1)

Dermatitis herpetiformis _subepidermal bullae._

Aetiology

An autoimmune disease asociated with gluten enteropathy and IgA in the skin. _in dermal perpulae_

Clinical features

Groups of small blisters or papulovesicles on an urticated background involving elbows, knees, buttocks, scalp and scapular areas. Intensely itchy excoriations rather than blisters are usually seen (Figs. 133, 134).

Treatment

Can be controlled by dapsone. A strict gluten-free diet.

Pemphigus _epidermal bullae._

Aetiology

Autoimmune disease directed against epidermal cells and intraepidermal cement.

Clinical features

A disease of the middle-aged, especially Jews. Widespread, erythematous erosions (or true blisters) on any area of the body (Fig. 135). Firm pressure on the surrounding skin will produce a sore. Mucous membranes are also involved. Tends to be fatal if left untreated.

Treatment

High doses of systemic steroids initially. Azathioprine as a steroid-sparing agent.

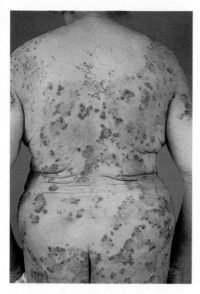

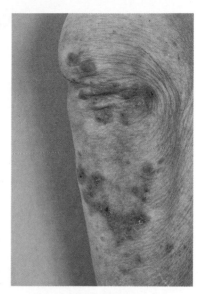

Fig. 133 Urticarial and annular lesions in dermatitis herpetiformis.

Fig. 134 The elbows are a characteristic site of involvement in dermatitis herpetiformis.

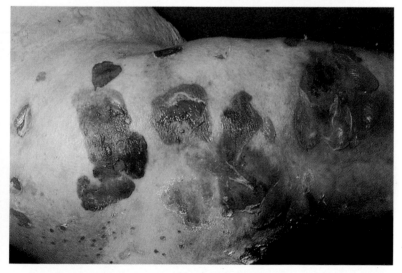

Fig. 135 Flaccid blisters and erosions (pemphigus).

Pemphigoid   sub epidermal lesions.

Aetiology

Autoimmune disease directed against the basement membrane of the skin.

Clinical features

A disease of the elderly. An urticated eruption develops initially (often on the limbs—Fig. 136), blisters usually appearing within a few days. Irritation can be intense. Blisters are large, thick-walled, tense and do not rupture easily (Fig. 137). Disease soon becomes widespread and symmetrical. Mucosal involvement relatively uncommon.

Treatment

High doses of systemic steroids initially. Lower maintenance dose for several months. Azathioprine as a steroid-sparing agent.

Cicatricial (mucosal) pemphigoid

Aetiology

Autoimmune disease closely related to pemphigoid.

Clinical features

A disease of the elderly. Blisters rupture to produce superficial erosions which heal with scarring. Mucous membrane of the mouth and conjunctivae are most frequently affected (Fig. 138), but the nose, throat, genitalia, anus and oesophagus can be involved. Scarring causes adhesions between conjunctival surfaces and scarring alopecia on the scalp.

Treatment

Systemic steroids may be required. Occular involvement must be treated by an ophthalmologist.

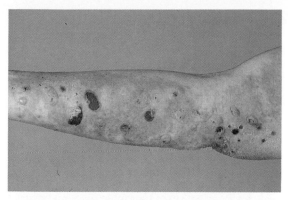

Fig. 136 Urticated and bullous lesions of pemphigoid.

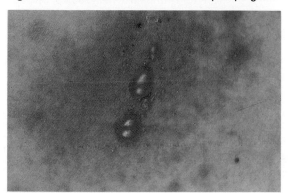

Fig. 137 Tense blisters in bullous pemphigoid.

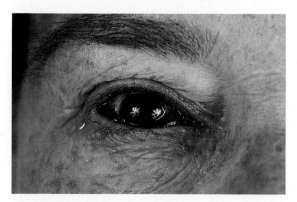

Fig. 138 Mucosal involvement in case of cicatricial pemphigoid.

Staphylococcus aureus

Clinical features

1. Boils/furuncles are Staph. hair follicle abcesses. Painful, red papules becoming pustular to heal with scarring. Atopy, diabetes and poor hygiene predispose. Patients may carry *Staph. aureus* in nose or perineum between attacks.
2. Folliculitis (Fig. 139) is a superficial Staph. infection of hair follicles. Small discrete pustules of beard, neck, scalp, buttocks and limbs.

Treatment

Antibiotics. Recurrent infections require swabs and appropriate antibiotics. Treat carriers (including family members) with antibiotic nasal cream and antiseptic baths/powder.

Streptococcus pyogenes

Clinical features

1. Erysipelas due to superficial infection with Strep. Tender, red and oedematous skin with a sharply demarcated, indurated edge.
2. Cellulitis (Fig. 140), a deeper Strep. infection with an ill-defined edge. Commonly involves face and legs. There may be associated lymphangitis and systemic toxicity. Diabetes, incompetent lymphatics and poor health predispose.

Treatment

Intramuscular penicillin.

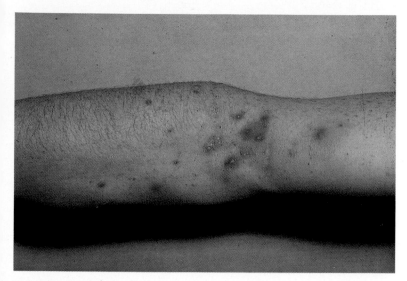

Fig. 139 Folliculitis.

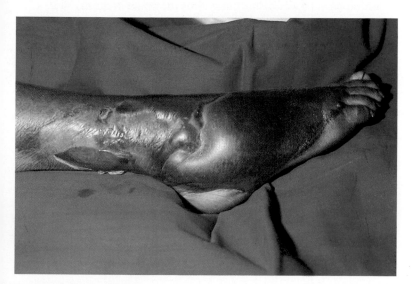

Fig. 140 Bullous cellulitis.

25 | Herpes Infection

Herpes simplex

Aetiology

Type I normally causes herpes labialis and type II genital infections.

Clinical features

Primary herpes simplex mainly occurs in children as stomatitis, fever and lymphadenopathy. Recurrent infections are characterised by *herpes labialis* ('cold sore') with small, closely grouped vesicles on an erythematous base. *Eczema herpeticum*—occurs in patients with atopic eczema and in the immunosuppressed.

Treatment

Cold sores—topical antiseptics, idoxuridine, or acyclovir. Oral acyclovir for severe/generalised herpes.

Herpes zoster

Aetiology

Varicella-zoster virus (dormant in dorsal root ganglion after childhood chickenpox).

Clinical features

Pain in the affected dermatome. After 1–3 days, clustered, red papules, becoming vesicular then pustular (Fig. 142). There may be fever, malaise and lymphadenopathy. Pain may persist for months. Involvement of ophthalmic division of trigeminal nerve may cause keratitis/blindness. Dissemination occurs in the immunosuppressed.

Treatment

As for herpes simplex. For post-herpetic neuralgia, analgesics, carbamazepine, tricyclic. antidepressants (or oral steroids, if given early).

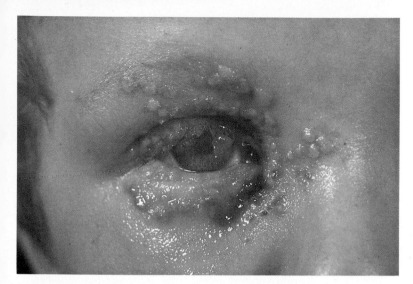

Fig. 141 Herpes simplex. A pustular and crusted eruption with fever, malaise and prostration.

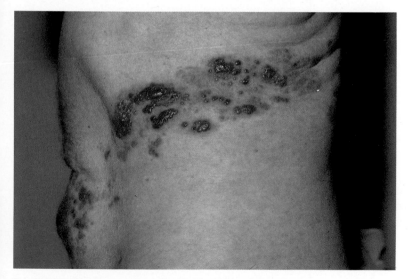

Fig. 142 Typical dermatomal distribution of herpes zoster.

Scabies

Aetiology

Sarcoptes scabiei var. *hominis*. Eggs are laid in epidermal burrows by the female acarus (mite). Overcrowding and sexual promiscuity predispose.

Clinical features

Pruritus is severe, intractable and worse at night; commencing about 2 weeks after the primary infection when the patient has developed hypersensitivity to the mite. Characteristic burrows (Fig. 143) are seen in finger webs and on flexor aspects of wrists, with characteristic papules on penis (Fig. 144) buttocks and around areolae. Vesicles may occur, but excoriations are more common (Fig. 145). Impetigo may coexist. Indurated, inflammatory nodules are sometimes seen on the scrotum and elsewhere. Lesions do not affect the head, except in infants, who often also have lesions around the umbilicus. The acarus can be demonstrated by scraping a burrow and examining the contents in 20% KOH under a microscope.

Treatment

Benzyl benzoate BP, 1% gamma benzene hexachloride and/or monosulfiram for children, applied on two consecutive nights following a hot bath. This should be combined with a change of contact clothing/bedding. All close contacts and all members of the household must be treated at the same time whether clinically affected or not.

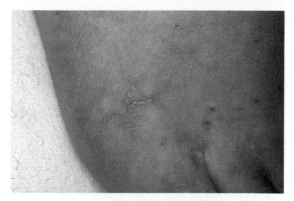

Fig. 143 Characteristic burrow of scabies.

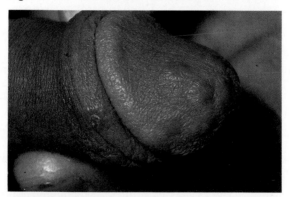

Fig. 144 Persistent penile papules (scabies).

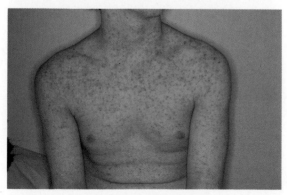

Fig. 145 Widespread pruritis rash of scabies.

Lice

Aetiology

Lice are translucent, wingless insects. Poor hygiene and crowded conditions predispose.

Clinical features

Head louse (p. 39).
Body louse. Asymptomatic pinpoint red macules. Pruritus, excoriations, papular urticaria and secondary infection follow, and hyperpigmentation in chronic cases (Fig. 146). Lice and eggs are found in the seams of clothing.
Pubic louse. Often transmitted by sexual contact. Intense pruritus of the pubic region. The eggs (nits) appear as grains of sand attached to the hair shafts.

Treatment

Remove nits with a fine-toothed metal comb. 0.5% Carbaryl/0.5% malathion lotions. Contacts must also be treated. Thorough disinfection of clothing.

Larva migrans

Aetiology

The larvae of various worms, e.g. *Angylostoma braziliense, Strongyloides stercoralis.*

Clinical features

The larvae penetrate the skin of feet, hands or buttocks. They migrate, producing intensely itchy, raised, red serpentine lines (Fig. 147).

Treatment

Local application of 10% thiabendazole suspension or oral thiabendazole.

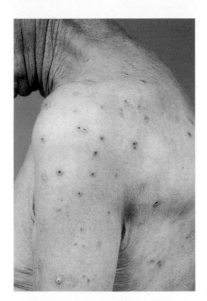

Fig. 146 Generalised excoriations (pediculosis corporis).

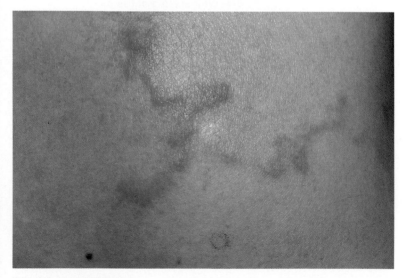

Fig. 147 Larva migrans.

27 | Fungal Infections (1)

Aetiology

Ringworm (tinea) infections enzymatically digest keratin. Obtain scrapings for microscopy and culture before beginning treatment.
1. Tinea pedis (athlete's foot) due to *Trichophyton rubrum, T. interdigitale* and *Epidermophyton floccosum.* Precipitated by communal showering, swimming pools and occlusive footwear.
2. Tinea manuum predominantly due to *T. rubrum.*
3. Tinea cruris caused by same as tinea pedis.
4. Tinea corporis by all types of ringworm.

Clinical features

1. Tinea pedis (Figs. 148, 150)—scaling, fissuring or irritation between 4th and 5th toes. May also be caused by bacteria, *Candida* or sweating. May produce erythema, scaling and occasionally vesicles/pustules on sole of foot.
2. Tinea manuum (Fig. 149)—characteristically unilateral with scaling of the palm. Exaggerated skin markings.
3. Tinea cruris occurs predominantly in young men. Well demarcated erythema and scaling in the groins with central clearing and 'active' edge (Fig. 151).
4. Tinea corporis—discoid, scaly areas which spread slowly with central clearing. Edge of lesion may be vesicular (Fig. 152).

Treatment

Topical antifungal agents e.g. Whitfield's ointment or imidazole creams/lotion, Castellani's paint for interdigital maceration. Griseofulvin 500 mg daily (with food) for 4–5 weeks may be necessary for *T. rubrum* or more extensive infections.

DERMATOLOGY

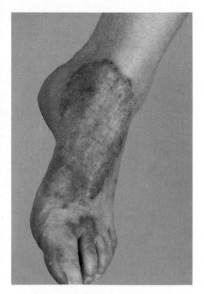

Fig. 148 Tinea pedis.

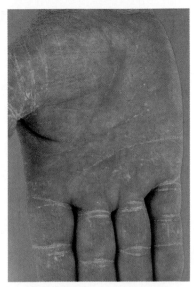

Fig. 149 Unilateral scaling of the palm (tinea manuum).

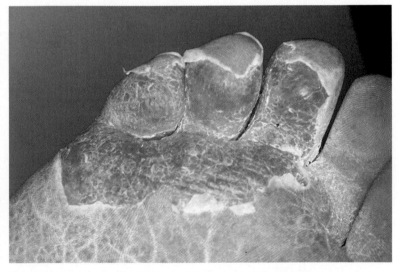

Fig. 150 Dermatophyte infection spreading out from the toes.

Tinea incognito

Aetiology

Ringworm infection modified by topical (or systemic) steroids (Figs. 148, 153).

Clinical features

The inflammatory response is suppressed by use of steroids. Itching and inflammation are reduced, the margins less distinct and scaling less apparent, yet slowly enlarging.

Treatment

Topical imidazole and oral griseofulvin. There may be some increase in inflammation on stopping the steroid.

Majocchi's ringworm granuloma

Aetiology

A foreign body granulomatous reaction due to folliculitis from *Trichophyton rubrum* (Fig. 153).

Clinical features

Predominantly in adults. An erythematous, scaly plaque on a limb studded with follicular pustules. Unilateral, but may spread to involve the whole limb.

Treatment

Oral griseofulvin 500 mg daily for 4–6 weeks.

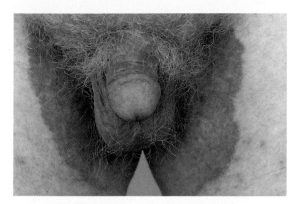

Fig. 151 Tinea cruris.

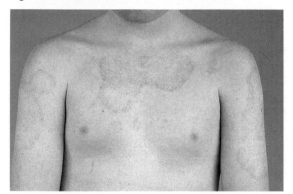

Fig. 152 Tinea corporis.

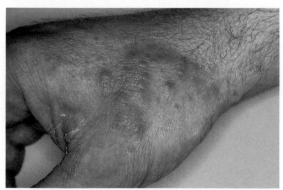

Fig. 153 Majocchi's granuloma.

Pityriasis versicolor (tinea versicolor)

Aetiology

Pityrosporum orbiculare.
Common in hot, humid environments.
Hyperpigmented or hypopigmented macules and fine superficial scales (Fig. 154).

Treatment

Selenium sulphide as body shampoo, topical imidazole creams. Tends to relapse. May take several months for normal skin colour to return.

Candidiasis

Aetiology

Candida albicans. Moisture, warmth, occlusion, antibiotics, steroid treatment, pregnancy and immunosuppression all predispose.

Clinical features

Erythema with scaling (Fig. 156) and papular or pustular satellite lesions at and beyond a well defined irregular edge, affecting skin folds esp. in obese patients (intertrigo). May be itchy or sore. *Napkin candidiasis* (p. 17).

Treatment

Nystatin or imidazole creams. Eradication of gut and vaginal yeast carriage.

Erythrasma

Aetiology

Diphtheroid *Corynebacterium minutissimum.*

Clinical features

Well demarcated brownish erythema in axillae, groins and toe webs with superficial scaling. Fluoresces coral-pink under Wood's light.

Treatment

Fucidin or imidazole cream; systemic erythromycin.

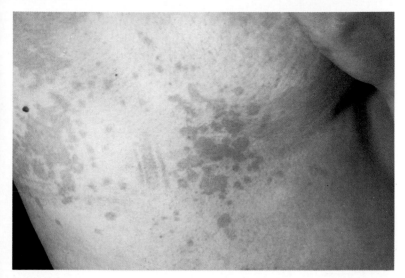

Fig. 154 Pityriasis versicolor. Well-demarcated rash common in hot, humid environments.

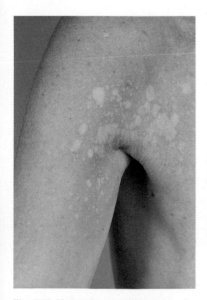

Fig. 155 Hypopigmented lesions of pityriasis versicolor. More conspicuous following sunbathing.

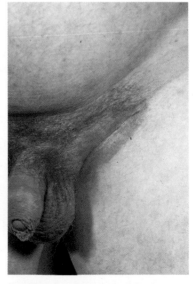

Fig. 156 Candidal intertrigo. Affects skin folds, especially in obese patients.

Seborrhoeic wart (basal cell papilloma)

Aetiology   Often familial.

Clinical features   Common in both sexes in middle life, usually on the trunk. Increase in number and size with age. Characteristically yellow-brown/black and greasy with a rough craggy surface (Fig. 157).

Treatment   Curettage (with application of superficial styptic). Cryotherapy.

Skin tag (fibroepithelial polyp)

Aetiology   Familial: obesity, pregnancy.

Clinical features   Multiple, soft, round and peduncular with a narrow base (Fig 158). Characteristically occur on the neck, axillae and groins.

Treatment   'Snip' and cautery. Diathermy.

Solar lentigo ('senile'/actinic lentigo)

Aetiology   Excessive exposure to sunlight.

Clinical features   A brown macule—often multiple—occurring on light-exposed skin of fair-skinned individuals. (Fig. 159).

Treatment   None. Cosmetics, cryotherapy, sunscreens.

Campbell de Morgan spot (cherry angioma; haemangioma)

Clinical features   Often familial, on trunk of middle-aged and elderly.

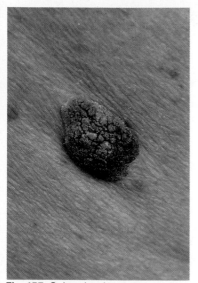

Fig. 157 Seborrhoeic wart. Differential diagnosis: malignant melanoma, pigmented BCC (when solitary and pigmented).

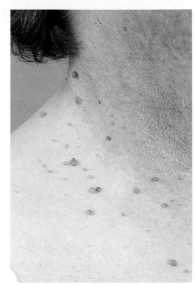

Fig. 158 Skin tags. Characteristically occur on neck, axillae, groin.

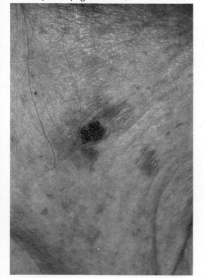

Fig. 159 Solar lentigo/seborrhoeic wart. Differential diagnosis: lentigo maligna.

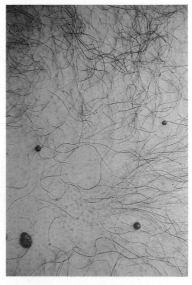

Fig. 160 Campbell de Morgan angiomas. Multiple, small bright red spots.

Solar keratosis (actinic keratosis)

Aetiology Chronic explosure to UVL.

Clinical features Commoner in the fair-skinned or expatriates, in middle to old age. Affects the backs of hands, forehead, scalp, temples, nose, cheeks and ears. Rough, adherent crusts on an erythematous base (Fig. 161).

Treatment Curettage and trichloracetic acid. Cryotherapy. 5-fluorouracil cream for multiple lesions.

Bowen's disease

Aetiology Previous exposure to UVL/or arsenic. Pre-invasive intraepidermal carcinoma.

Clinical features Appearing anywhere on the skin or mucosal surfaces as asymptomatic, erythematous, well-demarcated, scaly patches (Fig. 162). Ulceration suggests invasive growth.

Treatment Surgical excision, cryotherapy, 5-fluorouracil.

Keratoacanthoma

Clinical features Occurs in middle to old age, mainly on face or dorsum of hands. A flesh-coloured papule enlarges rapidly over 8–10 weeks with a central keratin-filled crater (Fig. 163). Spontaneous involution leaves depressed scar.

Treatment Surgical excision.

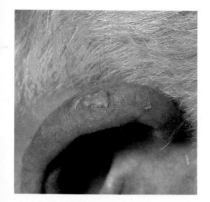

Fig. 161 Solar keratosis.

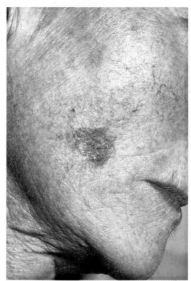

Fig. 162 Localised patch of Bowen's disease on the face.

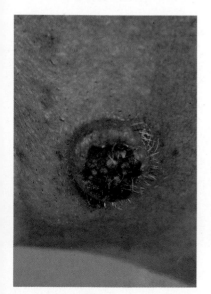

Fig. 163 Typical keratoacanthoma.

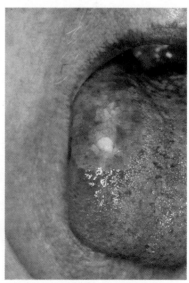

Fig. 164 Leukoplakia (carcinoma in situ). Well-demarcated white patches on tongue.

Basal cell carcinoma (BCC)

Aetiology

Chronic cutaneous sun-damage or exposure to arsenicals or radiotherapy.

Clinical features

Commonest cutaneous malignancy. Occurs in middle to old age, usually on the head and neck. Classically begins as a raised, pearly or translucent papule with telangiectasia, central ulceration and a typical rolled edge (Fig. 165). May be pigmented, multifocal or sclerotic/morphoeic (Fig. 167). Fibrosing or penetrating BCC may erode underlying tissues.

Treatment

Surgical excision. Radiotherapy. Curretage and cutery. Superficial multi-focal BCCs are sometimes treated with cryotherapy.

Squamous cell carcinoma (SCC)

Aetiology

Exposure to sunlight. Industrial carcinogens and longstanding ulcers also predispose.

Clinical features

May develop 'de novo' or in previously sun-damaged skin on a background of solar keratosis, Bowen's disease or leukoplakia. Begin as nodules on a firm indurated base, ulcerating as they enlarge (Fig. 166), commonly on the backs of hands and face, especially the lower lip and ear. Metastases are uncommon in the sun-induced type, but more frequent in 'de novo' SCC or on a background of Bowen's disease or leukoplakia.

Treatment

Surgical excision.

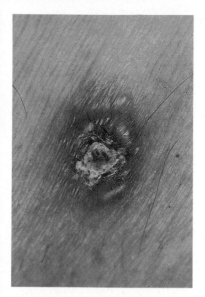

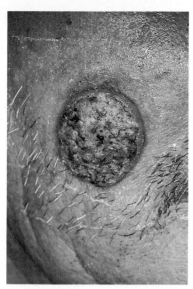

Fig. 165 Basal cell carcinoma with characteristic rolled, pearly edge.

Fig. 166 Squamous cell carcinoma of the face.

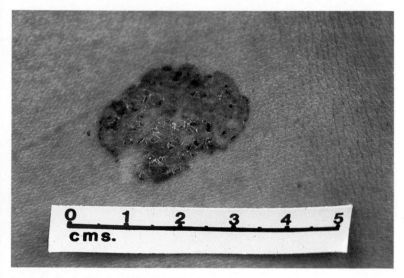

Fig. 167 Superficial multifocal pigmented BCC.

Lentigo maligna (Fig. 168)

Aetiology

Intraepidermal, pre-invasive, malignant melanoma.

Clinical features

Appears in middle to old age as a flat brown stain with an irregular, well-demarcated edge, slowly enlarging with variable pigmentation.

Treatment

Cryotherapy or superficial radiotherapy in the macular phase. Excision if small or nodular.

Malignant melanoma (Figs. 169, 170, 171)

Aetiology

Excessive exposure to sunlight.

Clinical features

Any 'new' mole or one which changes its character in adult life should be regarded as malignant melanoma until proved otherwise. Rapidly becoming the commonest form of cancer in the 20s–40s. Prognosis deteriorates rapidly and early referral is obligatory. Superficial spreading melanoma starts as a slightly elevated irregular brown or black patch.
Nodule formation indicates a vertically invasive stage. *Nodular melanoma* has a worse prognosis. Melanoma under the nail may be mistaken for subungual haemorrhage.

Treatment

Early wide excision with block dissection of lymph nodes if involved.

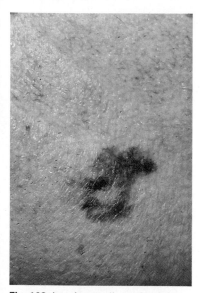

Fig. 168 Lentigo maligna. Nodular malignant melanoma may develop after many years.

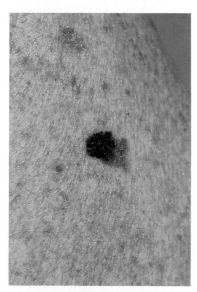

Fig. 169 Superficial spreading melanoma starts as slightly elevated irregular brown, or black patch.

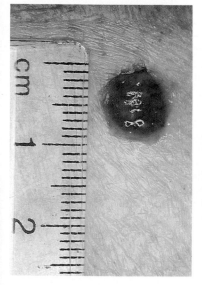

Fig. 170 Amelanotic (nodular) malignant melanoma.

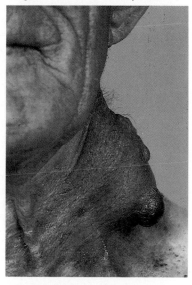

Fig. 171 Nodular malignant melanoma with lymphadenopathy.

33 | Contact Dermatitis

Aetiology

Irritant contact dermatitis (ICD) may be *acute* (strong irritants) or *cumulative* (mild irritants e.g. detergents/solvents), with progression from *irritant reaction* (dryness/chapping) to dermatitis. Atopy is a predisposing factor. *Allergic CD* (Figs. 172–175) is due to type IV (delayed) lymphocyte-mediated hypersensitivity. Common allergens include nickel, chromate, rubber, chemicals, medicaments and cosmetics (lanolin/preservatives/fragrance). Industrial allergens include epoxy, acrylate and phenol formaldehyde resins. Plant allergens include *Compositae*, *Primula obconica*, *Rhus* (poison oak/ivy) and various other woods and balsams. *Photo CD* may be allergic (e.g. musk ambrette), toxic (phytophotodermatitis) or simply light aggravated.

Clinical features

Hands and face, being in most contact with the environment, are the sites most commonly affected. The cause of the dermatitis may be obvious from the history, but patch testing is often necessary. Facial allergens may be volatile (airborne) or cosmetic. Medicament CD may be a complicating factor in stasis ulcers, chronic ear/eye disorders and in pruritus ani due to prolonged usage on damaged skin.

Treatment

Identify cause and advise on avoidance/ protection. Soap substitute, e.g. aqueous cream to clean/wash. 'Barrier' creams make hands easier to clean but afford no protection. Emollients. Topical steroids in strengths appropriate to severity of eczema. Rarely, systemic steroids. Antihistamines for symptomatic relief.

DERMATOLOGY

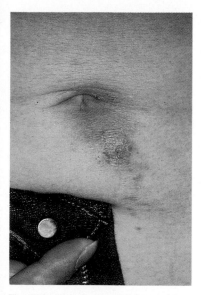

Fig. 172 Allergic contact dermatitis due to nickel jean stud.

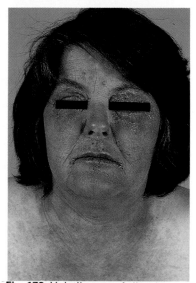

Fig. 173 Volatile type of allergic contact dermatitis due to phosphorous sesquisulphide in matches.

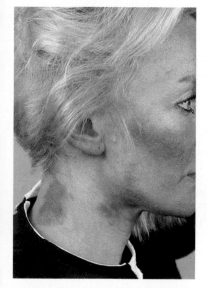

Fig. 174 Patchy erythema on neck due to nail varnish.

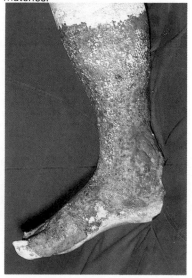

Fig. 175 Lower leg is an important site for medicament sensitivity.

Synonym	Hand dermatitis.
Aetiology	Constitutional or exogenous, frequently both, and impossible to differentiate on clinical appearances alone (Fig. 176). Atopics are more prone to irritant hand eczema.
Clinical features	*Constitutional patterns of hand eczema include*: Recurrent pompholyx; vesicular/hyperkeratotic hand eczema; hyperkeratotic hand eczema.

Exogenous patterns of hand eczema include:
Irritant patterns
a. 'Ring' eczema from wet work/detergents (Fig. 177).
b. 'Web' eczema/dorsum of hands from wet work.
c. 'Finger-tip' and 'palmar' patterns due to wet cloths, frictional factors, etc.
d. 'Patchy'/'discoid' patterns.

Allergic patterns
a. 'Non-specific'. Most cases, e.g. lanolin, perfumes, preservatives, etc. will be missed unless routine patch testing is performed.
b. 'Specific patterns', e.g. rubber glove dermatitis (Fig. 178), ring dermatitis, fingertip eczema.
c. Atopics may also develop type I *contact urticaria or protein contact dermatitis* from food handling and preparation.

Treatment   Identify the cause. Patch testing is helpful. Hand care advice, e.g. cotton-lined PVC gloves for wet work, frequent applications of emollients. Potent steroids with or without antibiotics for secondary infection. Atopics with a history of eczema should be given employment counselling.

DERMATOLOGY

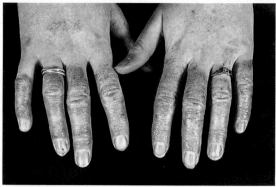

Fig. 176 Hand dermatitis: irritant and allergic factors frequently coexist.

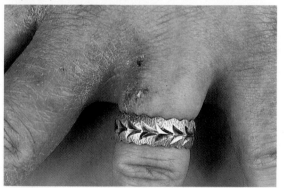

Fig. 177 'Ring' dermatitis—may be due to irritants, but occasionally associated with nickel allergy.

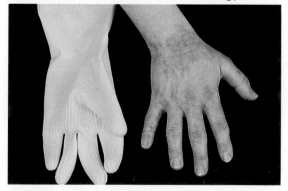

Fig. 178 Allergic contact dermatitis due to rubber gloves.

Pompholyx

Aetiology

A common form of endogenous eczema. May be a reaction to an active fungal infection of the feet. Ingested allergens (e.g. nickel in females) sometimes implicated.

Clinical features

A recurrent, intensely itchy, symmetrical eruption of the hands (and/or feet) with crops of clear vesicles on the sides of fingers and palms (Fig. 179). These may become confluent, producing large bullae. Secondary infection is common (Fig. 180). Skin subsequently becomes dry/fissured and desquamates.

Treatment

1. Frequent potassium permanganate soaks initially. 2. Potent topical steroids/antibacterial combinations. 3. Antihistamines for symptomatic relief. 4. Systemic steroids for severe attacks. 5. Antibiotics if secondary infection. 6. Treat athlete's foot if present.

Hyperkeratotic palmar eczema

Aetiology

Uncommon constitutional eczema not related to atopy. Factors include friction and underlying hyperkeratotic or psoriasiform tendency.

Clinical features

Usually affects middle-aged. Intensely itchy, hyperkeratotic patches of fissured eczema on palms. Rarely, there may be a few vesicles (Fig. 181).

Treatment

Potent topical steroids, antipruritic antihistamines, soap substitutes/emollients, tar, avoidance of friction, superficial RXT.

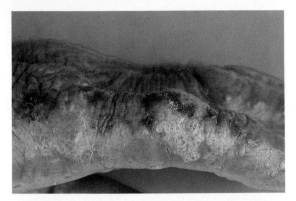

Fig. 179 Vesicular hand dermatitis (pompholyx).

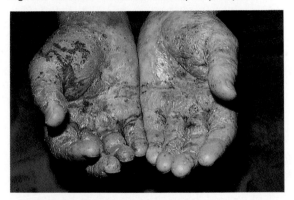

Fig. 180 Infected hand eczema.

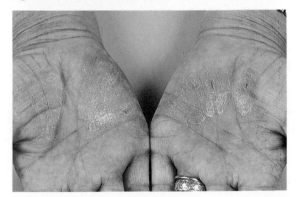

Fig. 181 Hyperkeratotic hand eczema.

Seborrhoeic eczema

Aetiology
Unknown. Not due to increased sebum production.

Clinical features
Infantile. 'Cradle cap' (p. 27); napkin (p. 19).
Adult. In young adults (usually men) commonly involves scalp, ears, eyebrows, eyelids, nasolabial folds, central chest and pubic area. Greasy scales on a background of erythema associated with generally greasy, easily irritated/intolerant skin (Fig. 182, 183). In the elderly, commonly intertriginous. Moist erythematous areas often with bacterial/candidal infection (Fig. 184).

Treatment
Soap substitutes. Weak topical steroids, steroid/antibiotic/antiseptic combinations; sulphur and salicylic acid cream, tar shampoos, steroid scalp applications.

Asteototic eczema

Aetiology
Reduced lipids and water binding capacity of the stratum corneum leads to drying/cracking of the skin. Aggravated by: excess washing, low temperature/humidity. Occasionally associated with malnutrition, general debility, diuretic therapy, myxoedema, renal failure.

Clinical features
Common in old age. Itchy, dry and scaly with reticulate cracks. Normally affects legs, but trunk and arms may be involved. Discoid eczema may coexist. Rarely, there may be an underlying malignancy.

Treatment
Emollients, bath oils, fewer baths. Weak topical steroids.

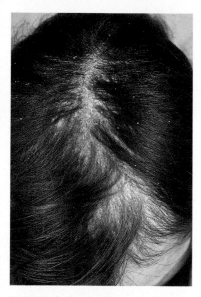

Fig. 182 Seborrhoeic dermatitis of scalp.

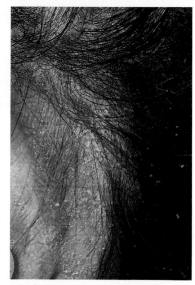

Fig. 183 Scalp margin and retro-auricular seborrhoeic dermatitis.

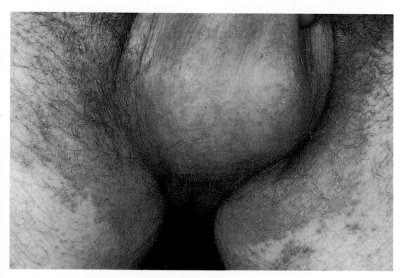

Fig. 184 Seborrhoeic dermatitis of the groin.

Discoid eczema (Figs. 185–187)

Synonym

Nummular eczema.

Aetiology

A constitutional pattern of eczema. Most cases occur in middle-aged men (executives) and stress, over-washing and low humidity, e.g. central heating, air-conditioning, car heaters, etc. may therefore be important. Characterised by well-demarcated coin-shaped areas of eczema, normally affecting the extensor surfaces of limbs but with subsequent explosive spread to a more generalised pattern of eczema. One or two solitary patches often pre-date the general eruption by some weeks or months. Pruritus may be intense. Lesions are often vesicular and exudative and may become secondarily infected. Often quite resistant to treatment.

Treatment

Soap substitutes. A reduction in bathing. Attempts to increase the humidity of surroundings. Emollients, oral antihistamines, potent steroids or steroid/antibacterial combinations, antibiotics. Systemic steroids may sometimes be required.

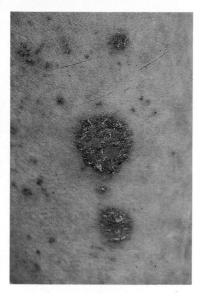

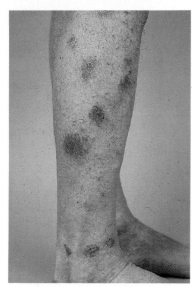

Fig. 185 Discoid eczema.

Fig. 186 Discoid eczema.

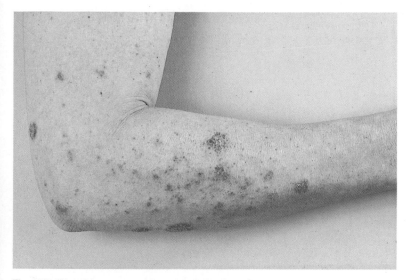

Fig. 187 Discoid eczema with secondary spread.

Stasis eczema (Fig. 175)

Aetiology

Venous hypertension resulting from deep vein thrombosis or familial valvular incompetence, poor tissue perfusion/oxygenation and incompetent, perforating veins.

Clinical features

Usually obese, middle aged women. Starts on the medial aspect of lower leg at site of perforating veins as stasis pigmentation. Oedema may become gross (elephantiasis nostras) (Fig. 188) or the leg may become progressively more fibrotic and sclerotic (Fig. 189) due to strangled microcirculation (atrophie blanche).

Complications

Ulceration, often following minimal trauma with the 'atrophie blanche' type leg. Secondary infection is invariable but normally only pathogenic bacteria (group A Strep. and *Staph. aureus*) require treatment. Streptococcal infection may cause cellulitis. Topical antibiotics frequently provoke allergic contact sensitisation.

Treatment

Weight reduction. Paste/compressive bandages. Support stockings when ulcers are healed. Rest with legs up. Oil helps scaly dry skin. Antiseptic solutions to clean ulcers, and simple dressings, e.g. paraffin gauze. Systemic antibiotics for secondary infection. Moderate strength steroids for eczema. Surgery for varicosities/incompetent perforators.

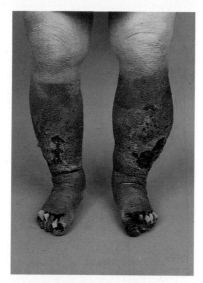

Fig. 188 Elephantiasis nostras.

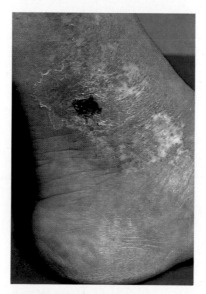

Fig. 189 'Atrophie blanche'.

Aetiology and clinical features

a. Secondary to venous hypertension (p. 123).
b. Secondary to arterial disease. Ulceration may follow arterial thrombosis, atherosclerosis, vasculitis or small vessel disease such as that associated with rheumatoid arthritis and diabetes. Peripheral pulsations may be diminished or absent and pain is a constant feature, especially at night or when dressings are too tight. The ulcers have a characteristic 'punched-out' appearance (Fig. 190) with a well-defined regular edge.

—Hypertension is an important complicating factor.

—Infection. Group A Strep. and *Staph. aureus* are the most important organisms.

—Neuropathic ulcers occur in diabetes (Fig. 192), alcoholics and in leprosy. They particularly involve the foot/lower leg. Secondary infection also often plays a part.

—Malignancy. A progressive, non-healing or 'atypical' leg ulcer should raise the question of a basal cell or squamous cell carcinoma.

—Other rare causes include sickle cell disease, spherocytosis, cryoglobulinaemia, tertiary syphilis (Fig. 191).

Treatment

In arterial disease, treatment is generally unsatisfactory since the underlying cause of the ischaemia is rarely reversible. Hypertension should be controlled, but N.B. betablockers reduce tissue perfusion. Appropriate antibiotics for secondary infection; intravascular abnormalities should be corrected where possible; adequate analgesia. Dressings should be simple and non-constricting.

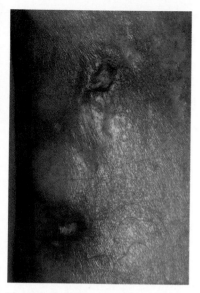

Fig. 190 Small punched out arterial ulcers.

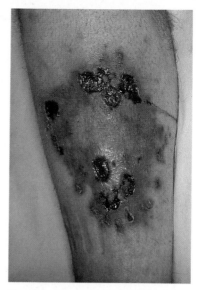

Fig. 191 Atypical ulceration (syphilis).

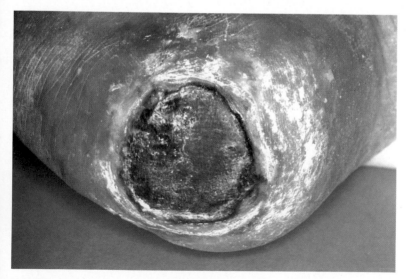

Fig. 192 Ischaemic neuropathic/pressure ulcer on heel of diabetic.

37 | Skin Manifestations of Internal Malignancy (1)

Acanthosis nigricans (Fig. 193)

Aetiology

Normally underlying adenocarcinoma of stomach, breast or lung, but benign and genetic forms also exist.

Clinical features

Thick, ridged, warty plaques give a velvety appearance in the axillae and groin. Heavily pigmented skin. (May antedate the clinical appearance of carcinoma by 3 or 4 years.) Benign forms occasionally occur both as genetic disease and as a complication of endocrine disease and obesity (Fig. 194).

Treatment

Treatment of the underlying condition may lead to resolution of the skin changes, but these may recur if the carcinoma spreads or metastasises.

Acquired icthyosis (Fig. 195)

Aetiology

Normally associated with underlying reticuloses, e.g. Hodgkin's disease or mycosis fungoides. Occasionally drugs, malabsorption and malnutrition.

Clinical features

Itchy, dry and scaly skin. There may be hyperkeratosis of the palms and soles.

Treatment

Treat the underlying disorder. Emollients, antipruritics and antihistamines.

Erythema gyratum repens, migratory thrombophlebitis (Fig. 196), and generalised pruritus are also in this category of disorder. Other recorded associations are less reliably attributed to underlying malignant disease.

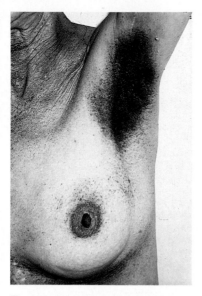

Fig. 193 Acanthosis nigricans in a patient with underlying malignancy.

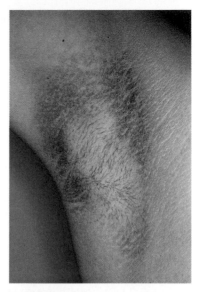

Fig. 194 Acanthosis nigricans (benign type).

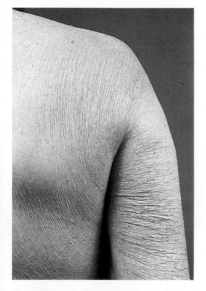

Fig. 195 Acquired ichthyosis with underlying lymphoma.

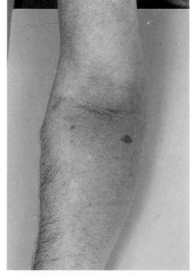

Fig. 196 Migratory thrombophlebitis.

| # Skin Manifestations of Internal Malignancy (2)

Dermatomyositis

Aetiology

An autoimmune disease. In those over 40, approximately half the cases will have an underlying carcinoma of lung, ovary, breast, uterus or stomach, but there is no such association in childhood.

Clinical features

A characteristic violaceous rash associated with myositis. There is also often a myopathy, and if this involves the respiratory muscles, the disease can be life-threatening. Other associations include arthralgia, Raynaud's phenomenon, fever and prostration. Calcinosis cutis is common in the childhood form. Erythema, fine scaling and telangiectasia affect the face with heliotrope discolouration of the upper eyelids (Fig. 197). Violaceous plaques occur over the knuckles, and cuticles become thick and ragged with prominent nail-fold telangiectasia (Fig. 198). Oedema of the hands and face is common. The rash may generalise.

Treatment

High dose steroids are required. Bed-rest. Splints and support for involved muscles and joints. General supportive treatment. Seek and treat the underlying carcinoma.

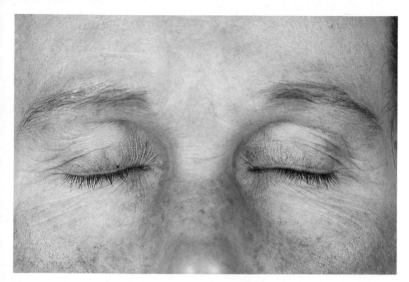

Fig. 197 Heliotrope discolouration of the eyelids in a patient with immune type dermatomyositis.

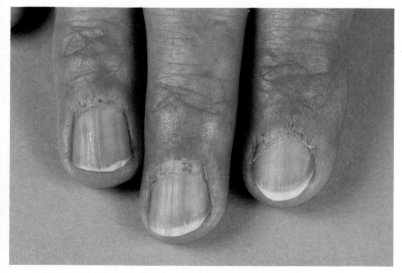

Fig. 198 Nail fold thromboses in a patient with dermatomyositis.

| **Autoimmune Diseases (1)**

Vitiligo

Aetiology

One of a group of organ-specific autoimmune diseases with antimelanocyte antibodies.

Clinical features

Well-defined oval or irregular depigmented areas (symmetrical and a few mm to several cm in size) affecting axillae, groins, genitalia, dorsum of hands and face (Figs. 199, 200). Hair in the affected areas may also become white. The involved skin tends to burn on sun exposure but is otherwise asymptomatic. Other organ-specific autoimmune diseases may coexist, e.g. thyroid disease, pernicious anaemia, diabetes melitus and alopecia areata in both patients and their families (Fig. 201).

Treatment

Not universally successful. Repigmentation may sometimes be induced with potent, topical steroids or PUVA. Cosmetic camouflage, sunscreens.

Halo naevus (Fig. 202)

Aetiology

Localised form of vitiligo.

Clinical features

An area of depigmentation surrounding a small pigmented cellular naevus. The central naevus usually disappears over several weeks and repigmentation may then occur or a leukodermic area persist. Some patients develop vitiligo.

Treatment

Sunscreens to protect vitiliginous area.

DERMATOLOGY

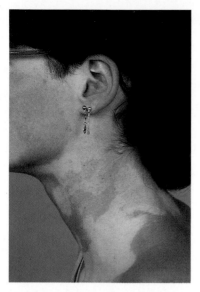

Fig. 199 Vitiligo contrasted with islands of normally pigmented skin.

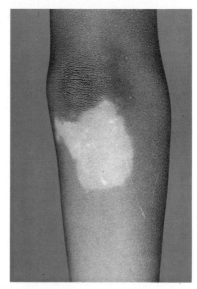

Fig. 200 Vitiligo in a dark skinned girl.

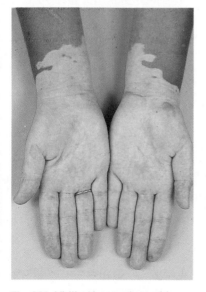

Fig. 201 Vitiligo in a patient with co-existent Addison's disease.

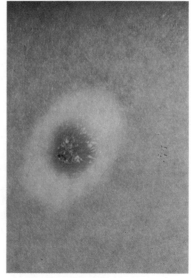

Fig. 202 Halo naevus.

Scleroderma

Synonyms Systemic sclerosis; acrosclerosis; morphoea.

Aetiology Unknown but thought to be autoimmune.

Clinical features

There are 3 principal types of scleroderma.

1. A *multisystem* disease (*acrosclerosis*) commonly affects women. Raynaud's phenomenon is a frequent presenting symptom. The skin of the hands and face is hard and tightly bound down. The fingers become tapered, flexed and shiny with loss of finger pulps (sclerodactyly) (Fig. 203). There may be nail-fold thromboses and fingertip ulceration. The face becomes mask-like with pinching of the nose and mouth. Telangiectasia and calcium deposits in the fingers are common. The gastrointestinal tract, liver, kidneys, joints and lungs may also be involved.

2. A more *progressive* form (*progressive systemic sclerosis*) affects both sexes equally. Morbidity and mortality are significant.

3. *Localised cutaneous scleroderma (morphoea)* normally affects young adults, women more than men. Ill-defined purplish, sclerotic plaques develop insidiously on the trunk and elsewhere, often symmetrically and progressing slowly over a matter of months/ years (Fig. 204). Special variants include 'coup de sabre' (parietofrontal), linear (Fig. 205) and generalised forms.

Treatment Always very disappointing. Steroids penicillamine, vitamin E and immunosuppressants have been tried.

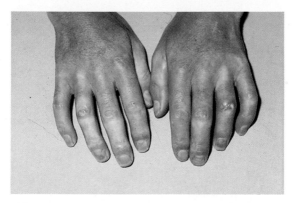

Fig. 203 Acrosclerosis.

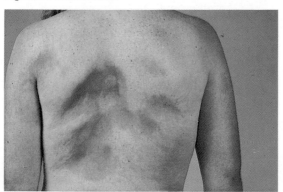

Fig. 204 Localised morphoea.

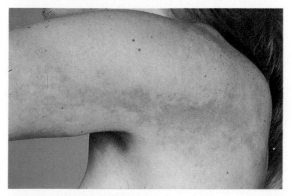

Fig. 205 Linear morphoea.

39 | Systemic Lupus Erythematosus (SLE)

Aetiology

Genetic predisposition to this and other autoimmune diseases. Virus infections and pregnancy may act as triggers. Drugs, e.g. hydrallazine and procainamide, can sometimes provoke an SLE-like syndrome.

Clinical features

A multisystem disease affecting women more than men. The skin, joints, kidneys, lungs, CNS and other organs may all be involved. Lymphopenia and thrombocytopenia are both common. There is often an element of photosensitivity or an eruption confined to light-exposed areas. This may be 'discoid-LE-like' (p. 81) or quite non-specific consisting simply of erythema or a discrete maculopapular eruption (Fig. 206). The classical pattern consists of a symmetrical patchy erythema, sometimes with scaling, telangiectasia and induration, occurring on the cheeks and bridge of the nose producing a typical 'butterfly' rash. The hands are also often affected and there may be vasculitis (p. 71), persistent non-itchy weals, livedo (Fig. 207) and chilblain-like lesions during the winter. Nail-fold infarcts and splinter haemorrhages occur in association with Raynaud's phenomenon (p. 133). There may be general symptoms including arthralgia, malaise and fever. Alopecia (Fig. 208) occurs in up to 50% of patients.

Treatment

Avoidance of exacerbating factors, e.g. cold and sunshine, and symptomatic treatment may be sufficient. Systemic steroids and immunosuppressants are usually required for more severe disease.

DERMATOLOGY

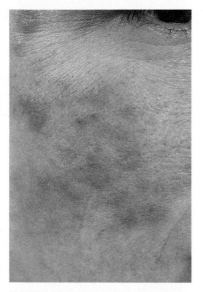

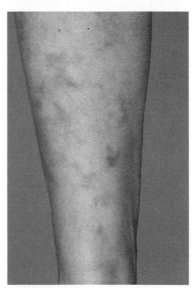

Fig. 206 Maculopapular-type LE of face.

Fig. 207 Livedo reticularis (SLE).

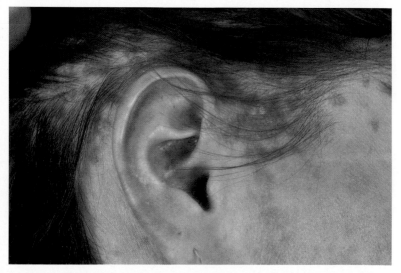

Fig. 208 Discoid LE-like lesions and scarring alopecia in a patient with SLE.

Adverse effect of topical steroids depend on (a) potency of preparation, (b) length of use, (c) site of use.

Aetiology

Steroids inhibit dermal collagen synthesis.

Clinical features

Atrophy. Thinning of skin occurs with long-term use of potent topical steroids. Affected areas are erythematous and fragile with telangiectasia (Fig. 209).

Striae. Commonly seen in axillae and groins; initial 'stretch marks' are purple and later become white (Fig. 210).

Purpura or bruising may arise following minimal trauma.

Tinea or *impetigo incognita.* Topical steroids may mask the characteristic appearance of fungal or bacterial infections (p. 103).

Perioral dermatitis. (p. 73)

Adrenal suppression. Application of potent topical steroids in large quantities (50–100 g/week) or under occlusion may lead to temporary suppression of pituitary-adrenal function. This is particularly important in young children.

Granuloma gluteale infantum. This condition occurs in infants a few months old who have received topical steroid applications for napkin rash. Small, often multiple, red-brown nodules develop anywhere within the napkin area. Nodules resolve slowly once the application of topical steroids is stopped (p. 18).

DERMATOLOGY

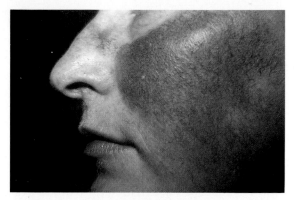

Fig. 209 Steroid-induced telangiectasia.

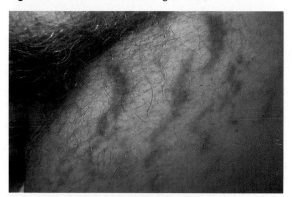

Fig. 210 Striae from topical steroids.

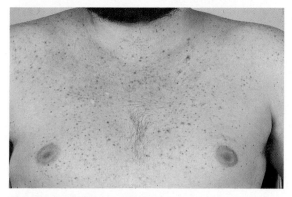

Fig. 211 Steroid acne folliculitis—a consequence of high dose systemic steroid therapy.

Sarcoidosis (Fig. 212)

Aetiology

Unknown. A multisystem, granulomatous disease.

Clinical features

Erythema nodosum. (p. 69)
Lupus pernio. Indurated, soft, blue-red plaques affect nose, ears, fingers, cheeks.
Papulonodular. Firm, blue-red papules, nodules or plaques affect the face, trunk and extensor surfaces of limbs. Annular lesions also occur.
Scar sarcoid. Existing scars may become infiltrated.

Treatment

Oral steroids if systemic symptoms warrant.

Annular erythema (Fig. 213)

Aetiology

Often idiopathic. Drugs, infections and carcinoma have been implicated. Variants include erythema chronicum migrans (tick bite), erythema gyratum repens (underlying carcinoma) and erythema marginatum (active rheumatic fever).

Clinical features

Small, pink papules enlarge slowly to form ring or polycyclic patterns with central clearing. May be solitary or multiple, lasting weeks/months.

Treatment

Symptomatic.

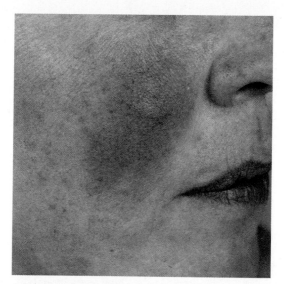

Fig. 212 Lupus pernio.

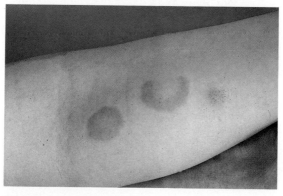

Fig. 213 Annular erythema.

Granuloma annulare (Fig. 214)

Aetiology

Unknown. May be associated with diabetes mellitus.

Clinical features

Commonly affects adolescents. Solitary or multiple firm, smooth, skin-coloured or violaceous papules on the dorsum of hands, fingers, ankles, elbows and elsewhere. Typically they progress into annular lesions. Most resolve spontaneously within 1–2 yr.

Treatment

None. Intralesional corticosteroids rarely.

Necrobiosis lipoidica (Fig. 215)

Aetiology

Unknown. Some cases associated with diabetes.

Clinical features

A reddish-brown, slowly enlarging plaque with a shiny, yellow, atrophic centre, classically involving the front of the shins. Lesions show telangiectasia and some eventually ulcerate. Differential diagnosis: granuloma annulare, basal cell carcinoma.

Treatment

Test for diabetes. Potent topical steroids are of limited value.

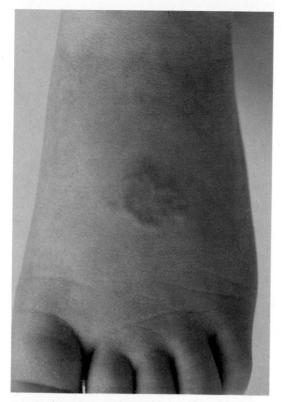

Fig. 214 Granuloma annulare.

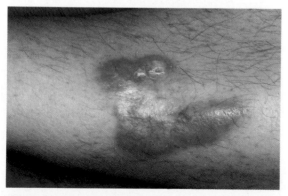

Fig. 215 Necrobiosis lipidoica.

Dermal Reactions (3)

Keloids/hypertrophic scars
(Figs. 216, 217)

Aetiology

Excess proliferation of dermal collagen. Risk increased with tension, infection or foreign material. Occasionally a family history. Hypertrophic scars commoner in Negroes.

Clinical features

Firm, raised, smooth, pink (or in Negroes brown) plaques or nodules develop 4–6 weeks after skin trauma, particularly on the upper back, shoulders, neck and presternal areas. Keloids tend to be irregular and to spread beyond the original injury.

Treatment

Intralesional steroids may help.

Xanthomatosis (hyperlipidaemias)

Aetiology

Localised cutaneous deposits of lipid. May be primary or secondary to diabetes, myxoedema, pancreatitis and nephrotic syndrome.
Xanthelasma. Symmetrical, firm, flat, yellow plaques affecting the upper and lower eyelids (Fig. 218). Usually no lipid abnormality; some have type II hyperlipidaemia with raised cholesterol levels and a positive family history.
Xanthomata. Firm, yellowish nodules over the knees, elbows, heels and buttocks (Fig. 219). Tendon xanthomas occur in types II and III hyperlipidaemia.
Eruptive xanthomata are small, yellow or red-brown papules occurring on the buttocks and extensor surfaces of the limbs; characteristic in type I and V lipidaemias but also common in type IV hyperlipidaemia.

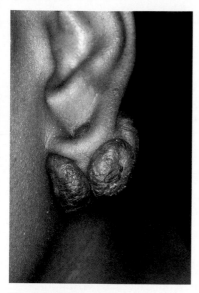

Fig. 216 Ear lobe keloid.

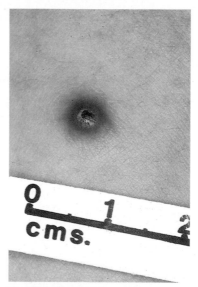

Fig. 217 Dermatofibroma—a localised fibrotic tissue response to insect bites.

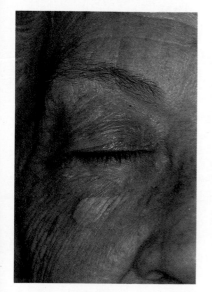

Fig. 218 Xanthelasma.

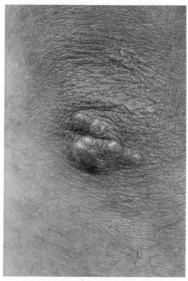

Fig. 219 Tuberous xanthoma.

Lichen planus (Fig. 220)

Clinical features

Mucous membrane lesions occur in 50% of cases but may occur in isolation. Candidiasis, secondary syphilis, leukoplakia must be differentiated.

Geographic tongue

Clinical features

Benign, inflammatory disorder of unknown aetiology, usually asymptomatic. Multiple smooth, erythematous patches migrate in a map-like pattern on the dorsum of the tongue.

Recurrent aphthae (Fig. 221)

Clinical features

Common disorder of buccal mucosae, tongue, and gingival folds. Small, erythematous pustules rapidly break down to form painful shallow ulcers which heal in 7–10 days.

Black hairy tongue

Clinical features

May follow antibiotics and cytotoxics. The elongated papillae ('hair') may be yellow-brown or black.

Leukoplakia

Clinical features

Small, discrete, white patches or more extensive, leathery plaques on an atrophic erythematous base. Tobacco smoking and recurrent trauma predispose. Risk of malignant change (p. 109).

See also Pemphigus (p. 87) (Fig. 222).

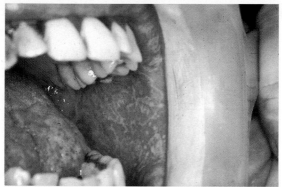

Fig. 220 Bluish-white lace-like striae of oral lichen planus.

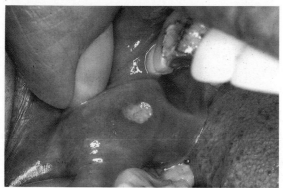

Fig. 221 Aphthous ulcer.

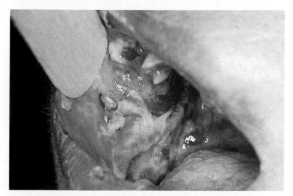

Fig. 222 Mucosal pemphigus.

Onychogryphosis (Fig. 223)

Aetiology

Age, trauma and ill-fitting shoes predispose.

Clinical features

Usually affects the great toenails. Hypertrophy progresses to typical 'ram's horn'.

Treatment

Regular chiropody.

Onycholysis

Aetiology

Causes include trauma (both physical and chemical), infection, psoriasis, eczema, poor circulation, photosensitivity to certain drugs, e.g. tetracyclines, and thyroid disease (Fig. 224).

Clinical features

Lifting of the nail plate distally. May develop secondary pseudomonas infection.

Treatment

Reduce trauma. Keep nails short and dry.

Onychomycosis (Fig. 225)

Aetiology

Usually trichophyton rubrum/mentagraphytes.

Clinical features

White or yellowish discolouration. The nail becomes thickened with subungual hyperkeratosis, splinter haemorrhages and onycholysis.

Treatment

Griseofulvin—6 months for finger nails, 12—18 months for toenails.

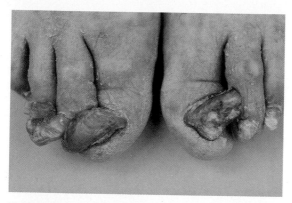

Fig. 223 Onychogryphosis.

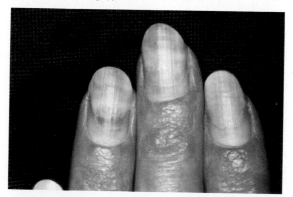

Fig. 224 Onycholysis.

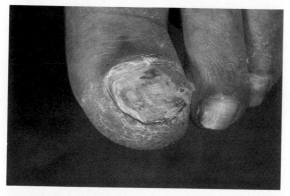

Fig. 225 Onychomycosis.

Nails in Dermatological Conditions

Psoriasis (Fig. 226)

Clinical features

The nails may be involved in the absence of psoriasis elsewhere. Pitting, onycholysis, subungual hyperkeratosis, yellowing/thickening and splinter haemorrhages. Treatment is generally unrewarding.

Lichen planus (Fig. 227)

Clinical features

Nail changes can occur in the absence of lesions elsewhere. Increased longitudinal striations of nail plate, producing ridging and splitting. Nail plate becomes thinned and may progress to atrophy with scarring or even permanent destruction. The cuticle may grow over the base of the nail and attach to the nail plate.

Treatment

Rarely, intralesional or systemic steroids.

Alopecia areata

Clinical features

The nail plate becomes dull and roughened, with small, fine, regular pitting. There is no specific treatment.

Eczema (Fig. 228)

Clinical features

Nail changes can occur in any type of eczema, but are more often seen in atopic eczema. Several changes occur including: coarse pitting, transverse irregular ridging, and shedding.

Treatment

Treatment of the underlying eczema.

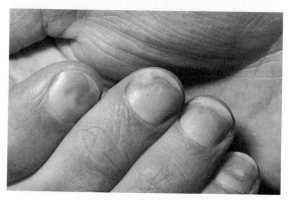

Fig. 226 Onycholysis and wax spots (psoriasis).

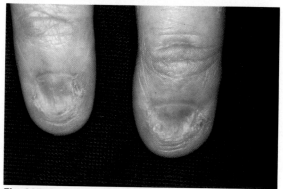

Fig. 227 Atrophy and scarring of the nail plate (lichen planus).

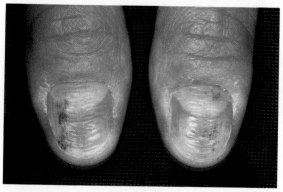

Fig. 228 Transverse ridging of the nails (eczema).

Lichen planus (p. 57)

Clinical features

Characteristic mauve papules with fine lacework of white striae occur on the penile shaft, glans, and prepuce in men (Fig. 229), and in women, on the inner surface of the labia. Annular forms may also occur. Affected areas are frequently pruritic. May occur with no evidence of lichen planus elsewhere. Treatment is symptomatic.

Lichen sclerosis et atrophicus

Clinical features

Uncommon (? autoimmune) disease mainly affecting women. Ivory-white or violaceous areas on the perianal and vulval regions with 'cigarette paper' atrophy. There may be follicular plugging, erosions and fissuring. In males, the glans penis and foreskin may be involved, leading to phimosis or meatal stricture (Fig. 230). Dyspareunia, soreness and pruritus often cause distress. Potentially premalignant.

Treatment

No specific therapy known. Hydrocortisone/antiseptic creams for symptomatic relief. Potent topical steroids for phimosis or meatal strictures; 2% testosterone proprionate is also said to help. Surgery.

Psoriasis (p. 47)

Clinical features

Well-defined smooth, erythematous plaques on genitalia (Fig. 231). Important to differentiate from erythroplasia of Querak (Bowen's disease).

Treatment

Mild–moderate steroid/antibacterial creams.

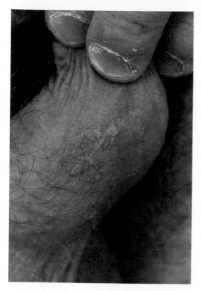

Fig. 229 Annular lichen planus.

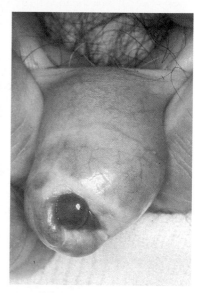

Fig. 230 Meatal phimosis due to lichen sclerosis et atrophicus.

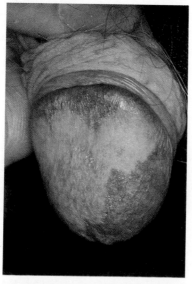

Fig. 231 Psoriasis of glans penis.

46 | Hair

Alopecia areata

Aetiology

An organ-specific autoimmune disease.

Clinical features

Characterised by sudden hair loss in discrete, discoid patches (Fig. 232). Spontaneous regrowth often occurs in those with limited disease, although the new hair may initially be white. Occasionally progresses to involve the whole scalp (Fig. 233) or body. At the periphery of patches, diagnostic exclamation mark hairs are seen (Fig. 234). There may be associated fine pitting of the nails.

Treatment

Reassurance and wait for spontaneous regrowth. Topical or intralesional steroids, topical irritants (e.g. Dithranol), ultraviolet light/PUVA and contact sensitisation may help. Topical 1% minoxidil solution may help those with localised patches. Wigs.

Scarring alopecia (p. 82, 136)

Aetiology

A result of destruction of hair follicles in, e.g. discoid lupus erythematosus, lichen planus, scleroderma, burns, infections, radiodermatitis.

Clinical features

Atrophic scalp with absent hair follicles. Once hair is lost regrowth never occurs.

Management

Treatment of the underlying condition. Wigs.

DERMATOLOGY

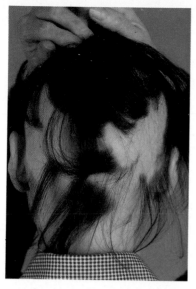

Fig. 232 Alopecia areata.

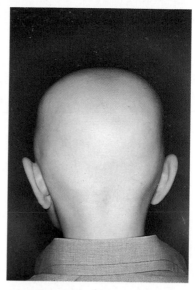

Fig. 233 Alopecia totalis.

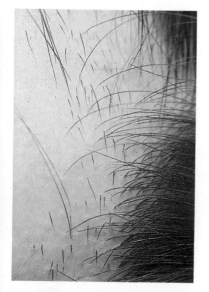

Fig. 234 Exclamation marks hair in active alopecia areata.

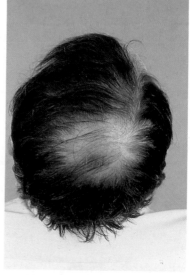

Fig. 235 Bi-temporal recession and early androgenic pattern hair loss.